The Double Contrast Examination of the Colon Experiences with the Welin Modification

Archiv und Atlas der normalen und pathologischen Anatomie in typischen Röntgenbildern

Fortschritte auf dem Gebiete der Röntgenstrahlen und der Nuklearmedizin
Diagnostik, Physik, Biologie, Therapie

Ergänzungsbände:
Band 105

Herausgegeben von
W. Frommhold, Tübingen
und P. Thurn, Bonn

Unter Mitwirkung von
G. Breitling, Tübingen
R. Glauner, Stuttgart
R. Glocker, Stuttgart
K. zum Winkel, Berlin

Georg Thieme Verlag
Stuttgart

The Double Contrast Examination of the Colon Experiences with the Welin Modification

by Sölve Welin and Grethe Welin

141 Illustrations, 5 Tables

Thieme Edition
Publishing Sciences Group, Inc.

Prof. Dr. med. CARL-SÖLVE WELIN
Dr. med. GRETHE WELIN

Malmö Allmänna
Sjukhus/Sweden

ISBN 3-13-522101-6

For Distribution in USA and Canada,
Publishing Sciences Group, Inc., 162 Great Road,
Acton Massachusetts 01720

ISBN 0-88416-088-2 LCCCN 75-37198

Preface

The pathologic processes of the large intestine of greatest interest to roentgenologists originate in the mucosa. It is therefore only natural that endeavors have been made to obtain as detailed a picture of the mucosa as possible; I modified the double contrast method to meet this requirement. Since the middle of 1953 this modification has been used routinely in the Department of Diagnostic Roentgenology, Malmö General Hospital. By the time of my retirement in the middle of 1970 more than 50,000 examinations had been performed with the method, and the number has increased considerably since then. This book is based on my own and my co-workers' experiences during those 17 years.

The differential diagnosis between Crohn's disease and ulcerative colitis was developed and formulated in cooperation with Grethe Welin, former assistant doctor in the Department of Diagnostic Roentgenology, Malmö General Hospital, now Director of the Department of Diagnostic Roentgenology, Diakonissestiftelsen's Hospital, Copenhagen.

Contents

1 History

It was not long after the discovery of roentgen rays that endeavors were made to examine the gastrointestinal tract roentgenographically. As early as 1896 Becker tried to fill the stomach and bowel in guinea pigs with a metal salt (a lead solution) and was thus able to demonstrate various segments of the gastrointestinal tract. He pointed out the possibility of producing a roentgenogram of the human stomach and thought it should be possible to use this method for demonstrating fistulae. In the same year an American, Cannon, visualized various parts of the digestive tract of a goose with the aid of heavy metal salts. In 1901 Hildebrand, using bismuth as contrast medium, obtained a roentgenogram of the human transverse colon and reported to the Medical Society in Hamburg that he used the same method for demonstrating other parts of the intestinal tract. He added: "With this method (bismuth) it would probably be possible to demonstrate and locate intestinal stenosis due to carcinoma". The idea had occurred to Hildebrand while examining a patient who had taken bismuth: several small shadows were seen in the patient's colon.

Two years later, in 1903, Williams wrote that the position and outline of the colon could be demonstrated either by rectal infusion of a fluid containing a radiopaque substance such as bismuth or by insufflation of the colon with air.

Work in this field was continued by Rieder: in a lecture delivered to the Gesellschaft für Morphologie und Physiologie in Munich in 1904 he reported that he had roentgenographically studied the topography of the gastrointestinal tract in a living person. For this purpose he had administered bismuth orally and rectally. He also stated that the bismuth enema produced a more detailed roentgenogram, stressing that the method had been used previously by Stegman and Schüle.

An article describing in detail how to demonstrate the site and extent of a tumor after infusion of bismuth was published by Schenk in 1908. He was convinced that a wider application of this method would sometimes reveal operable tumors of the colon.

At a roentgenologic congress in Detroit (1910) Haenisch stated that a bismuth enema was far better than a bismuth meal in examination of the colon, although the latter method was more physiological. He added that the bismuth enema could be given under fluoroscopic control, and presented a number of roentgenograms of various lesions of the colon.

Thereafter it was generally recognized that roentgenograms obtained after enemas were superior to those obtained after meals, especially since the barium enema had been introduced in 1914. Since that time many enthusiastic articles have been published describing the results obtained with this method.

However, it was gradually realized that the results obtained with barium enema were not satisfactory, especially in the diagnosis of neoplasms. Small tumors were not discovered and even larger ones could be overlooked when situated in unfavorable positions. Endeavors were therefore made to improve the method. Knothe (1927), for example, reported that he used as small an amount of barium as possible and that the bowels were emptied before roentgenography. The roentgenograms thus obtained showed very fine details of the internal mucosa. Knothe regarded this as an obvious improvement.

A report by Kalkbrenner (1928) soon followed stating that he had obtained better pictures of the outline of the mucosa with thorium dioxide sol than with barium. He published some roentgenograms far better than those obtained with a conventional barium enema. Gilbert and Kadrnka (1933) tried

Umbrathor, which tended to adhere to the wall of the colon and was therefore preferable to the rapidly sedimenting barium.

This procedure was then widely adopted, but since it often proved difficult to obtain satisfactory adhesion of the preparation to the wall of the intestine, it was abandoned until it was later taken up again in America.

Thus, in 1946 Hamilton reported that he had tried Sackett's method, which consisted of the addition of tannic acid to the barium enema. This produced a better mucosal pattern in the post-evacuation films. The method was introduced in many quarters, and in 1950 Christie et al. reported that they had carried out 4,225 such examinations. They claimed that any lesion of 1 cm or larger could be seen and that they were thus able to demonstrate certain functional and organic changes of the colon which they had never been able to visualize previously.

They concluded that the use of tannic acid had proved a valuable complement to previous methods of examining the large intestine, because a uniform coating of the mucosa of the completely contracted colon was thus obtained. However, the late Professor Weber – former director of the roentgen department of the Mayo Clinic – was not especially optimistic and claimed that the addition of tannic acid to an opaque enema did not result in a more satisfactory examination.

In 1933 Ledoux-Lebard and Garcia-Calderon attacked the problem from a different angle; they proposed the use of a semitransparent contrast medium but this was expensive and produced very poor fluoroscopic images. The conclusion they drew was that a semitransparent study must be supplemented by a second enema of fully opaque barium.

In 1936 Rigler and Eriksen advocated overexposed films to demonstrate polypoid growths of the stomach, and at about the same time Gianturco employed a high voltage technique in the investigation of the large bowel – at first 100 kV, but later 120 kV. He also used a semi-opaque barium suspension. He believed that the high voltage technique would visualize not only polypoid growth of the colon but also other lesions somewhat more often than other methods. He first published his experiences with this method in 1950, and three years later described a series of 1,552 patients thus examined, demonstrating polyps in 2.7 percent.

The method was taken up by Jarre, and by Fiegel and Fiegel in Detroit, in 1961. They used a large compression pad and made several spot roentgenograms. They postulated that this technique made the double contrast method superfluous.

The double contrast method was originated by Fischer, a German surgeon, in 1923. He used barium and air simultaneously, pointing out that it was thus possible to obtain an outline of the intestine even when several loops were superimposed on one another and that even small growths were demonstrated, which might have been concealed by a solid column of barium. In Europe the method attracted little interest at first. However, further developments were stimulated by Dr. Kirklin – former director of the department of diagnostic radiology at the Mayo Clinic – who came to Europe in 1928. He visited Fischer and was greatly impressed by the potentialities of Fischer's examinations. Returning home Kirklin relayed his impression of this technique to Harry Weber, one of his associates. After two years' perseverance Weber succeeded in improving the double contrast technique in such a way that it consistently produced diagnostic roentgenographs. Thus in 1930 the American version of the double contrast examination was established, although for some reason few roentgenologists were able to perform it. Consequently it was adopted only very slowly by other clinics.

At the annual meeting of the Radiological Society of North America in 1949, Bell presented a paper on "General Considerations in the Roentgen Examinations of the Large Bowel". At the same meeting Morson delivered a lecture entitled "Double Contrast Examination of the Colon" (not published). Afterwards Garland asked: "Must one put 95 to 98 patients to the discomfort, expense and hazard of double contrast studies for the sake of the other 2 to 5? We doubt that the answer is 'yes'. It is our impression that double contrast studies are indicated in only about 10 percent of persons coming to the average radiologist for colon examination."

By 1953 Gianturco had become more cautious; he felt that the double contrast method was an interesting and beautiful procedure with which it was possible, under favorable conditions, to demonstrate even very small polyps. He even went as far as to claim that under certain conditions the brilliance of such films is second to none. But he added, how often are the conditions so favorable?

Two years later De Peyster and Gilchrist were also somewhat sceptical – although they succeeded with the double contrast method. They felt that the high voltage technique with diluted contrast medium produced still better results.

On the other hand, several authors held quite a different opinion. In 1952 Stevenson, for example, stated that this is the most reliable diagnostic procedure for detecting early carcinoma of the colon, although 15 percent of the examinations will fail to show a good double contrast in the cecum and portions of the ascending colon due to insufficient barium/air balance. Douglas (1953) felt that with this technique small lesions situated above rectoscopic level could be recognized better than with any other method.

In the same year Moreton proposed that the ideal routine study in all cases of colonic disease should include double contrast enema, either as a supplement to the plain barium enema examination or as the primary procedure.

Thus, although many roentgenologists found that the double contrast method was an obvious improvement for the demonstration of small changes, it was not adopted as routine procedure. Several authors again emphasized that superior diagnostic information was obtainable from postevacuation films. In 1954 Robinson postulated that the postevacuation film was superior to the double contrast method for diagnosing a tumor, and Marshak and Lindner wrote as recently as 1972 that the roentgen changes in Crohn's diesease of the colon are usually better demonstrated in the barium-filled colon than in air-contrast studies. They added: "The evacuation film is often superior to both the barium- and the air-filled colon study for determining the extent of the disease, the presence of skip lesions and the detection of tiny ulcerations and nodular mucosal alterations, so typical of Crohn's disease of the colon. Of course it is not necessary to restrict the examination to one procedure. Optimal evaluation is achieved by utilizing the filled colon, double-contrast and postevacuation films. For those primarily interested in beauty, the air study technique is suggested."

In my experience – based on more than 50,000 examinations since our technique included also a postevacuation film in order to compare the two methods – postevacuation films are superior to those obtained with the conventional barium enema. The method, however, still had serious disadvantages, and our investigation showed that the results were not as good as with my modification of the double contrast method. In postevacuation films small polyps are, as a rule, concealed and even if they should by chance be detected, these films will tell nothing about their base. Nor were the results satisfactory in patients with inflammatory mucosal changes.

One cannot control or master the rate of emptying of the intestine. The large intestine often empties far too much, so that not enough contrast medium remains to form a coating on the mucosa. In other cases emptying may be incomplete; then too much contrast medium will be left and the mucosal pattern cannot be evaluated.

The results obtained with the "mucosal relief method" in the early 1950s did not meet the new requirement of a refined roentgen diagnosis. Clinicians wanted roentgenologists to diagnose polypoid neoplasms as small as a few millimeters in diameter. At that time it was postulated that carcinoma of colon and rectum often developed from the small polypoid lesions. I therefore tried to find better ways of cleaning and preparing the intestinal wall for the double contrast method. I felt that it must surely be able to detect even very small changes in the colon. If the large bowel can be evacuated of all solid and fluid contents and if an even, extremely thin contrast coating can be created on the wall of an intestine highly distended by air, then any change in the mucous membrane or polypoid indentation must be caused by a process involving the intestinal mucosa.

It was soon realized that if the method was to be used routinely, four conditions had to be satisfied:

First of all, perfect cleaning is essential.

Secondly, the intestinal mucosa must be prepared so as to permit the adhesion of an extremely thin and even contrast coating of the intestinal wall.

Thirdly, one must be able to regulate evacuation, so that the intestine empties itself satisfactorily and the various stages of the examination can be carried out at very short intervals to avoid any unnecessary waiting time.

Finally, it should not be necessary for the patient to be in the x-ray room for more than 20 to 25 minutes.

After these conditions had been met the examination was used routinely from the spring of 1953. Between July 1, 1953, and July 1, 1970, when I retired, more than 50,000 examinations were performed in the Department of Diagnostic Roentgenology in Malmö. The number has since increased. In my opinion, this modification is clearly superior to all other x-ray examination methods because it reveals extremely important details of the mucosa of diagnostic value; details which are not demonstrable by any other method hitherto known.

2 The Examination

To obtain the best results from the examination the following five prerequisites must be satisfied:

1. A clean colon.
2. An adequately prepared intestinal wall.
3. An excellent barium suspension.
4. A well insufflated bowel.
5. A fine roentgen technique.

A Clean Colon

One of the most troublesome factors in roentgenology of the large bowel is the presence of feces and mucus, which interfere with the interpretation of the roentgenograms. This is especially disturbing at double contrast roentgenography for which the bowel must be completely clean.
The degree to which the bowel can be cleaned depends on three factors, viz. the sort and amount of food the patient eats the day before the examination, the cleansing effect of the fluid introduced into the intestinal canal, and the motility of the intestine.
The *food* should not contain non-absorbable substances. Patients should therefore be instructed to eat a diet poor in roughage, such as boiled chicken, fish, soup, raw or boiled eggs. The food should be well minced. On the other hand, all high-roughage food such as bread, potatoes, rice, vegetables, fruit and fat should be avoided. This diet should be ordered for at least one day before the examination.
The *fluid* may be given orally or rectally. Formerly the fluid was given as an enema, usually containing more than one constricting agent. The enema method is most effective when the last enema is given immediately before the roentgen examination and by experienced assistants.
In 1961 Garland Brown described an entirely new method – a hydration method. The patient drank a large amount of fluid – water, milk or juice, for example, – at least 1.5 liters to influence the consistency of the intestinal contents.
With regard to *motility* one may use various stimulating agents. The most widely used stimulant is castor oil, which contains a substance that irritates the mucosa and forces the intestinal contents quickly through the small intestine into the colon, which is afterwards flushed clean by an enema. In recent years tablets and suppositories containing substances causing contraction of the bowel have been used, but have not produced satisfactory results.
The advent of contact laxatives implied a great advance. These laxatives are pure crystalline compounds insoluble in water. They are not absorbed in the bloodstream, and they have no undesirable effects on the blood picture, the function of the kidneys or the liver. The exact mode of action of the drugs is not yet properly understood, but they are believed to act directly upon the mucosa of the large bowel through a local reflex. These laxatives have little or no action on the small bowel.
Contact laxatives fall into two groups according to their mode of action. Their chief representatives are dioxyphenylisatine and diacetoxyphenyl-pyridyl-methane. Dioxyphenylisatine acts primarily directly on the annular and longitudinal muscle fibers with consequent increased tonicity of the intestinal wall, while the other preparation diacetoxyphenyl-pyridyl-methane mainly produces continuous contractions from the ascending colon down to the sigmoid.
In Malmö we started to use Exacton, a German laxative, which belongs to the latter group. It produced contractions of the intestine almost immediately, but in our opinion the effect was not always satisfactory. The bowel was never really clean, and the contrast coating of the mucous membrane was not always as good as one might

wish. Therefore, after extensive clinical tests tannic acid was added to both the cleansing enemas and the barium enemas.
Tannic acid has been used in enemas for centuries. In roentgenography it has been used even since the 1930s, especially in the United States, and in 1936 Thomas estimated that 25 percent of all barium enemas then given in the United States contained tannic acid.
The addition of tannic acid had several advantages:

1. It is sufficiently irritating to stimulate contractions of the entire colon and acts as a powerful purgative.
2. It is an astringent and inhibits the secretion of mucus as well as the transsudation of fluid into the lumen of the colon.
3. Tannic acid solution is viscous and therefore causes the barium to adhere to the bowel wall, giving it a good even coating without artefacts, bubbles or flaking.
4. Owing to a continuous contraction of the entire colon from the cecum to the rectum the residual intestinal contents, especially gas, are forced from the colonic tract.

According to some American investigators, there is no other procedure that will expel gas from the colon with such force and completeness as a tannic acid enema.
The concentration of tannic acid recommended for use in enemas varies between 0.25 and 3 percent. Too low a concentration will have no effect, and too high a concentration will cause excessive abdominal cramps. If an overdose is given, it is a potent hepatotoxin with a direct effect on the liver cells.
Some workers allege that infusion of 0.5 percent tannic acid solution is a satisfactory, reliable, harmless, simple and non-expensive preparation of the patient. Other workers regard 1 percent as the optimal concentration. In our experience 0.25 percent is enough for the cleansing enema and 0.5 percent for the barium enema.
The addition of tannic acid to the contact laxative – Bisacodyl – was an important advance. It meant that the colon could for the first time be properly cleansed and the intestinal mucosa prepared in such a way that a thin and even layer could be obtained on the wall of the colon, adequately distended by insufflation of air. This enabled visualization of even small details and a considerable refinement of the diagnosis.
It would, of course, be a great advantage if both ingredients – Exacton (Bisacodyl) and tannic acid – could be used in a single preparation containing amounts that had proved suitable in clinical practice, namely 3 mg of diacetoxyphenyl-pyridyl-methane and 5 grams of tannic acid. By special treatment the otherwise pratically insoluble laxative, Bisacodyl, was made readily dispersible in the presence of tannic acid. The preparation – Clysodrast – is now commercially available as a powder that is readily soluble in water.*
Clysodrast is so fast-acting that it is possible to use the double contrast method as a routine procedure. In our experience Clysodrast is an ideal adjuvant with which the colon can usually be effectively emptied and cleansed, but it can sometimes cause symptoms such as weakness and nausea and occasionally acute abdominal pain. These symptoms are generally only transient. When assessing the optimal amount of tannic acid that should be included in the preparation, large doses were used, and then the symptoms were more pronounced, and on a few occasions – in the examinations of epileptics – even cramps occurred.
In 1964 the U.S. Food and Drug Administration in Washington prohibited the use of tannic acid in enemas in man. The Clysodrast preparation was therefore withdrawn from the market, although clinical trials had shown that in the amounts included in the preparation tannic acid was not noxious. After further clinical and experimental investigations this has been confirmed and at the request of American roentgenologists the use of the preparation was again permitted (1972). The Food and Drug Administration stated, however, that the preparation is contraindicated in patients under the age of 10 years and that the total dosage of Clysodrast for any complete colonic examination, including the cleansing enema, should not exceed 7.5 g. No more than 10 g of Clysodrast should be administered to any individual within a 72-hour period. Today each packet contains only half of the former dose.
When I was informed that Clysodrast had been withdrawn from the market I began work with my wife, Dr. med. Grethe Welin, and a chemist, Torwald Åberg, of AB Ferring in Malmö to try to find a new substitute for the preparation. After various experiments we found that Cascara

* AB Ferrosan, Malmö, Sweden

sagrada was a contact laxative, a hitherto unknown fact. We began to use this preparation instead of Clysodrast. In our experiments we also tried to find a substitute for the cleansing enema, since it was very inconvenient for ambulant patients.

In 1968 Garland Brown visited us in Malmö and demonstrated his method, which was quite a new approach to the preparation for barium enema examinations. Brown claimed that in most of the earlier methods the patient was left in a varying degree of dehydration. The result of the dehydration is colonic absorption of water from the barium enema mixture, which increases the concentration of the barium sulphate suspension. Therefore, it is most desirable to have complete hydration of all patients prepared for barium enema examination. Brown's procedure results in a more consistent state of full hydration of the patients.

According to Brown, preparation of the patients should begin approximately 18 hours before the scheduled time of barium enema examination. For an examination that begins at 8 a.m. the preparation begins the day before at noon. The patient is given a low residue, non-fat lunch. He is hydrated throughout the day by drinking at least one full glass (240 cc) of water every two hours from noon until midnight. For supper the patient is given a clear liquid diet at 5 p.m. At 8 p.m. 340 cc of cold magnesium citrate solution are administered. This is followed at 10 p.m. by 3 Dulcolax pills with a full glass of water. At 7 a.m. the following morning he drinks one-and-a-half glasses of water and inserts a 10 mg Dulcolax suppository into the rectum. By 8 a.m. the patient is ready for examination, having had one or more final bowel movements resulting from the suppository.

In 1961 Brown had prepared approximately 2,500 patients by this method and a preliminary analysis of 200 of these patients indicated that the procedure was excellent in 95 percent. A transient mild nausea was reported by about 20 percent, but most stated that this was not incapacitating and the procedure was without detrimental side effects.

After Brown's visit we began to try his method and modified it somewhat. Since my retirement these trials have been continued under the supervision of my successor, Professor Boijsen and Dr. Jan Erik Rosengren and have resulted in the so-called Cascara-Salax method, which is described in a later section of this book. Most patients tolerate the new cleansing method but it has the side-effects attending all forms of severe laxation.

No serious side-effects have so far occurred, but owing to the effect of magnesium sulphate the method should not be used in patients with impaired renal function.

The Coating

A factor of great importance is the coating of the intestinal wall. If the coating is good, the mucosa can be thoroughly studied and extremely small lesions, if any, can be detected.

The intestinal mucosa must therefore be prepared in such a way as to permit adhesion of an extremely thin and even coating on the intestinal wall. The coating should not be interrupted or uneven.

Clysodrast serves this purpose well, but in order to check the action of the secretory glands still more, since a mucous layer may not only conceal the small pathologic changes but also impair adhesion of the contrast medium, the patients are medicated with atropine before the examination.

On arrival in the x-ray department the patient is given 1 mg of atropine by mouth. This inhibits the intestinal secretion and mitigates the pain frequently arising as a natural consequence of the pronounced contractions produced by the laxative agent in the enema. Later it mitigates the distress of bowel distension following the insufflation. Pretreatment with atropine has the additional advantage of offering protection against hypotensive episodes which may sometimes occur in connection with enemas in patients receiving treatment with ganglionic blocking agents. In children the dose of atropine should be reduced according to age and weight (Table 1).

Table 1. Premedication with Oral Atropine

Age in years	Dose (mg)
3 to 6	0.25
6 to 9	0.50
9 to 12	0.75
over 12	1.0

Another point requiring attention is the local water supply. The water used should be hard (without any additive to make it soft), since we have found that otherwise bubbles form during insufflation of the colon. If the water is not suitably hard, water soluble calcium salt should be added. Kernig uses four tablespoonfuls of calcium lactate per liter of barium mixture to reduce the formation of bubbles.

Barium Suspensions

Various types of barium suspension are available for double contrast roentgenography, and each x-ray department should itself decide which one is most suitable.

A poor suspension can cause trouble. Some form large bubbles, some flocculate badly and cause artefacts simulating lesions (Fig. 1). This so-

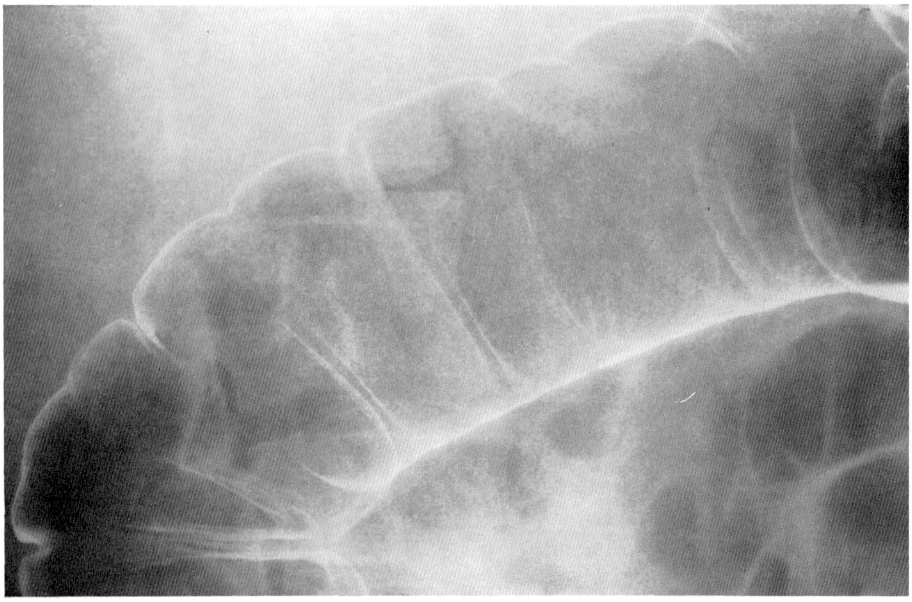

Fig. 1 ♂ 23 years:
a) X-ray 12/5/72: normal mucosal pattern.

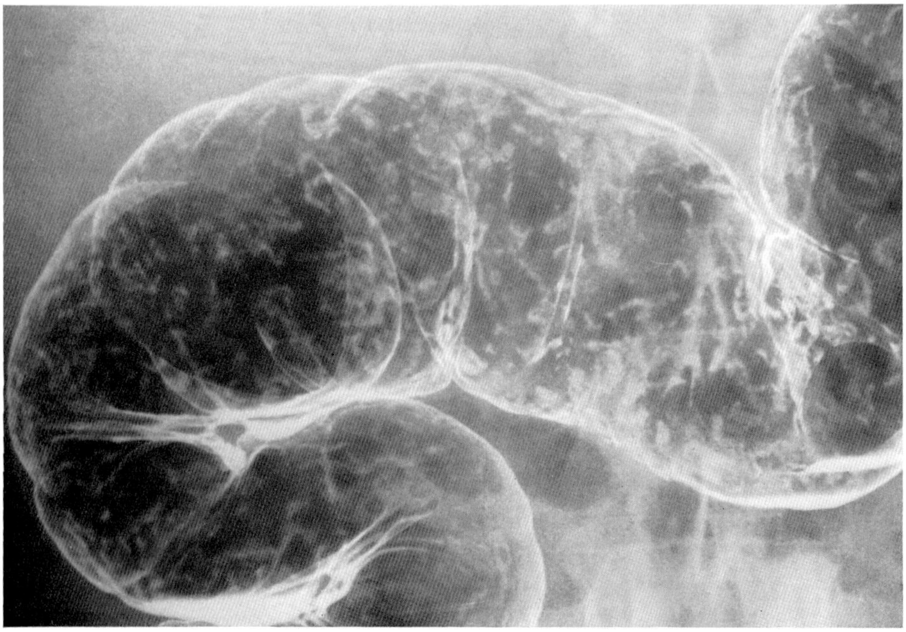

b) X-ray 10/5/72: flocculation.

called flocculation is probably due to the amount of citrate added to the contrast medium. The more citrate, the less flocculation, since the citrate binds fluid in the contrast layer and prevents it from being absorbed by the intestinal wall.

Serious endeavors have been made to improve the contrast medium. The quality of the medium depends mainly on three properties.

First, the size of the particles. This should not be larger than 0.5 to 1 μm. It is thus a question of very small particles and they should be of very uniform size to produce an electrostatic tension between them. These particles will then repel one another and, according to some authors, give an almost colloidal suspension. No such suspension is obtained with barium sulphate. Some manufacturers therefore add citrate ions to a concentration of about 0.5 percent.

The second point is the addition of an adhesive such as CMC (carboxymethyl cellulose), carraginate or gum arabic to secure good adhesion of the contrast medium to the mucosa. Such a coating of contrast medium ought to be very thin so as not to conceal small lesions in the mucosa.

The third point to be considered is the concentration of the barium sulphate. It should be proportional to the amount of adhesive in order to secure satisfactory radiopacity of the contrast medium. In the examination of the large intestine with the double contrast method 0.65 g barium per ml of contrast medium is suitable. It is also very important to use the same concentration of suspension from day to day; its density must be kept constant. To control the concentration of the barium we use Philip's Barium Specific Gravity Tester. This is adjusted to 6.5, which is not the true specific gravity.

Insufflation

Adequate insufflation, usually with 1,800 to 2,000 cc, is essential. It is performed in the ordinary way with Higginson's syringe. If the patient cannot retain the contrast enema or the air, a ballooned tube is used.

Roentgen Technique

The roentgen technique must be good and the images should be well defined. We therefore use a film-focus distance of 1.5 m when possible and a tube with a fine focus. High kV technique is suggested (approximately 90 to 100 kV) with 200 to 300 mA. Since practically no peristaltic waves occur in the distended intestine a long film-focus distance and a fine focus will produce a detailed roentgenogram.

3 Preparation of the Patient

The preparation of the patient varies considerably from one x-ray department to another. Earlier the procedures were not satisfactory and often constituted a stumbling block. It was widely believed that all attempts to obtain a really clean intestine were doomed to fail, but with techniques described below it is possible to clean the intestine thoroughly in about 90 percent of the patients and of the remaining 10 percent only a few require re-examination.

I. The Clysodrast Method

1. The day before the examination the patient is kept on light and easily digestible low-residue food, so there will be no cellulose particles present in the colon. Two tablets of a contact laxative are given at noon and two at 6 p.m., or 30 ml of castor oil at noon. Castor oil is usually more effective than the tablets.

In the evening – about 8 p.m. – the patient is given a water enema, and we have found that this enema is very important. In ambulant practice we sometimes use a plastic bag, containing sulphate magnesia, a wetting agent and a citrate buffer. After dilution with 2 l of water it is ready for use, and its pH is 4. This preparation is an isotonic solution and is therefore not absorbed by the colon.

2. The following morning the patient may have a cup of coffee or another drink and some toast. On arrival at the x-ray department he is given 1 mg of atropine by mouth. At the earliest half an hour after the administration of atropine the patient is given a simple water enema, to which has been added one package of Clysodrast. This enema, which consists of 2 l of water is given in the x-ray department by specially trained assistants. We have found it extremely important that this cleansing enema should *not* be given in the ordinary ward, *not* at the ordinary outpatient department, *not* at home, but *by the staff of the x-ray department,* so that one is absolutely sure that it is properly done. The enema should be given slowly with the patient first on the left side, then prone, then on the right side, and finally supine. The patient must receive the entire amount, and should be encouraged to retain the enema. In this way the cleansing enema routinely reaches the cecum.

3. After rest and evacuation of this cleansing enema the patient receives the barium enema containing so much Clysodrast that the concentration of tannic acid in the enema is 0.5 percent. The barium enema should reach the splenic flexure but no further.*

The colon is afterwards insufflated with the patient first prone and afterwards in the right lateral position, the supine position and finally in the left lateral position.

The contrast medium should by then have reached the cecal pole. Then the requisite x-ray pictures are taken.

II. The Cascara-Salax Method

When using the Cascara-Salax method the patient should be given the contents of a packet of Salax dissolved in a glass of water and 2 tablets of cascara sagrada at 8 a.m. the day before the examination. The mixture should be taken at breakfast. Salax includes magnesium sulphate, the major part of which remains in the intestine,

---

* If a postevacuation film is required for studying the mucous membrane and for making sure that the colon is clean, patients may evacuate this enema. After this a roentgenograph is taken, and the patient is given another barium enema, which should not go beyond the splenic flexure.

thereby increasing the osmotic strength of the intestinal contents which thus retain their fluid consistency right down to the rectum. The anthroquinone glucosides in the cascara sagrada thereby stimulate intestinal peristalsis with good emptying effect.
At noon, the patient is allowed to eat food with little roughage such as eggs, fish and meat, to drink a glass of water containing the dissolved contents of a new package of Salax and to take a further 2 Cascara tablets. He is thus not allowed to eat food from the plant kingdom – bread, potatoes or fruit. All forms of fat should be avoided.
The patient should then drink at least one glass of fluid – water, milk or juice – every hour until he retires for the night.
He may have a meal at 6 p.m. composed of such products as those mentioned above.
On the morning of the examination the patient is given no breakfast, but he may drink as much as he wishes.
Half an hour before the roentgen examination 1 mg atropine should also be given by mouth.
For ambulant patients this preparation is usually sufficient, but in elderly, bedridden or constipated patients the preparation should be supplemented by a cleansing enema on the morning of the examination. The enema should contain 1.8 gm cascara sagrada. After evacuation of the enema the roentgen examination should be performed in the usual way. If desired a postevacuation film may be obtained (see footnote p. 10).
Most patients tolerate this preparation well, but side-effects usually of the type following any form of severe laxation, may occasionally occur. No serious side-effects have so far occurred, but owing to the magnesium sulphate the method should not be used on patients with impaired renal function.

4 The Roentgen Examination

At examination roentgenograms may be obtained in those projections considered desirable or in standard projections according to a special schedule, in order to secure the best possible images of each part of the bowel. With the latter method the roentgen dose to which the patient is exposed is much smaller than that with the former technique.

In the latter case we used the following projections:

1. Three exposures of the rectum and sigmoid with the patient prone, a frontal view and two oblique lateral views with the patient turned 30–45° to the right and to the left. (Film size 24 × 30 cm). Figs. 2–4.
2. Lateral view of the rectum and the lower part of the sigmoid with the patient in the left lateral position. Film size 24 × 30 cm. Fig. 5.

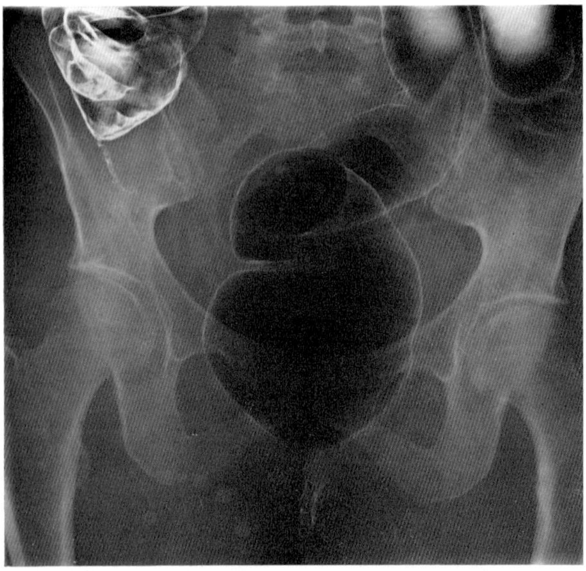

Fig. 2 Standard projection. Frontal view. Patient prone.

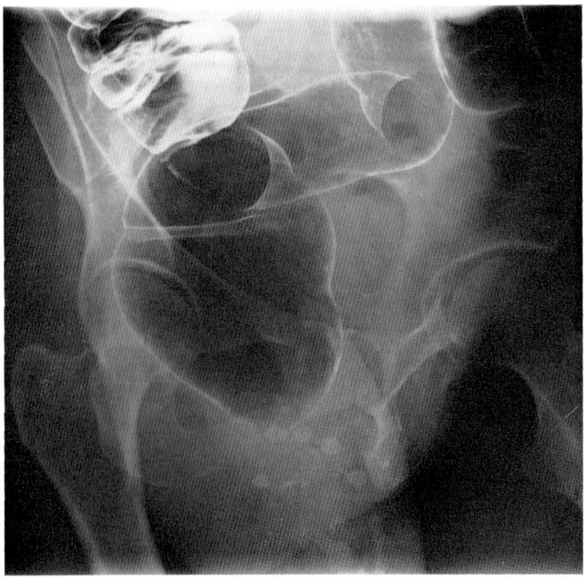

Fig. 3 Standard projection. Right anterior oblique. Patient prone.

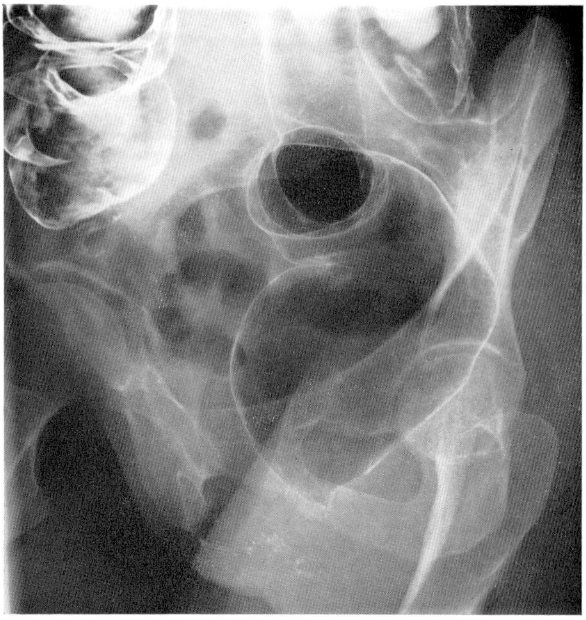

Fig. 4 Standard projection. Left anterior oblique. Patient prone.

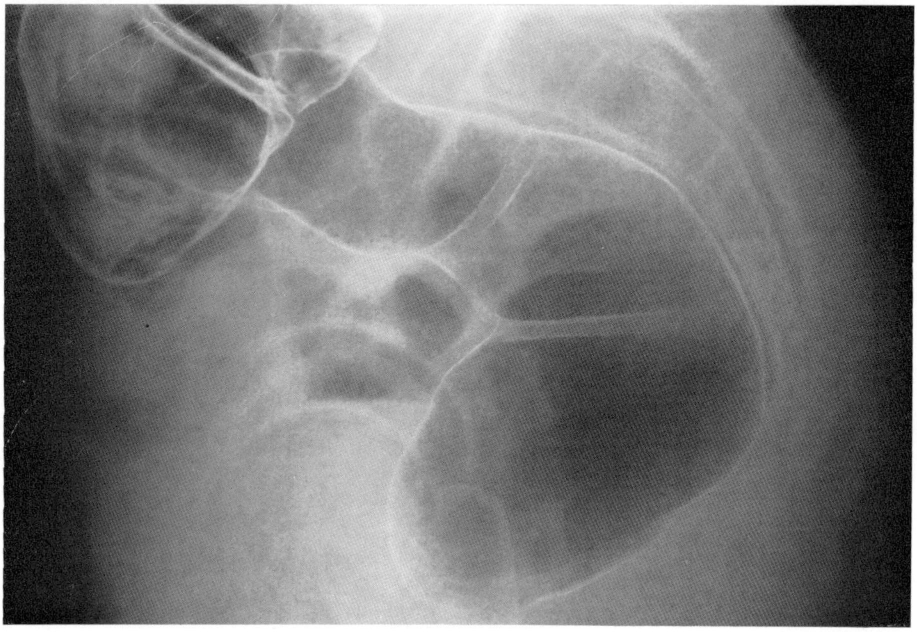

Fig. 5 Standard projection. Lateral view.

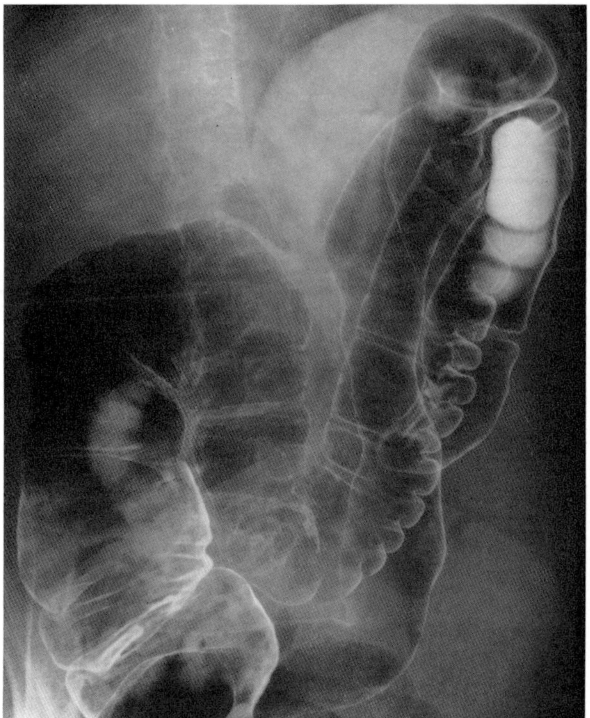

Fig. 6 Standard projection. Right posterior oblique. Patient supine.

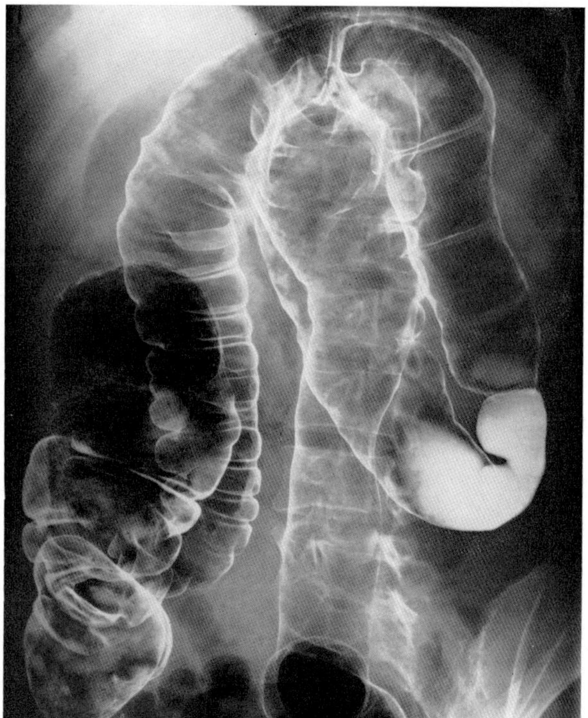

Fig. 7 Standard projection. Left posterior oblique. Patient supine.

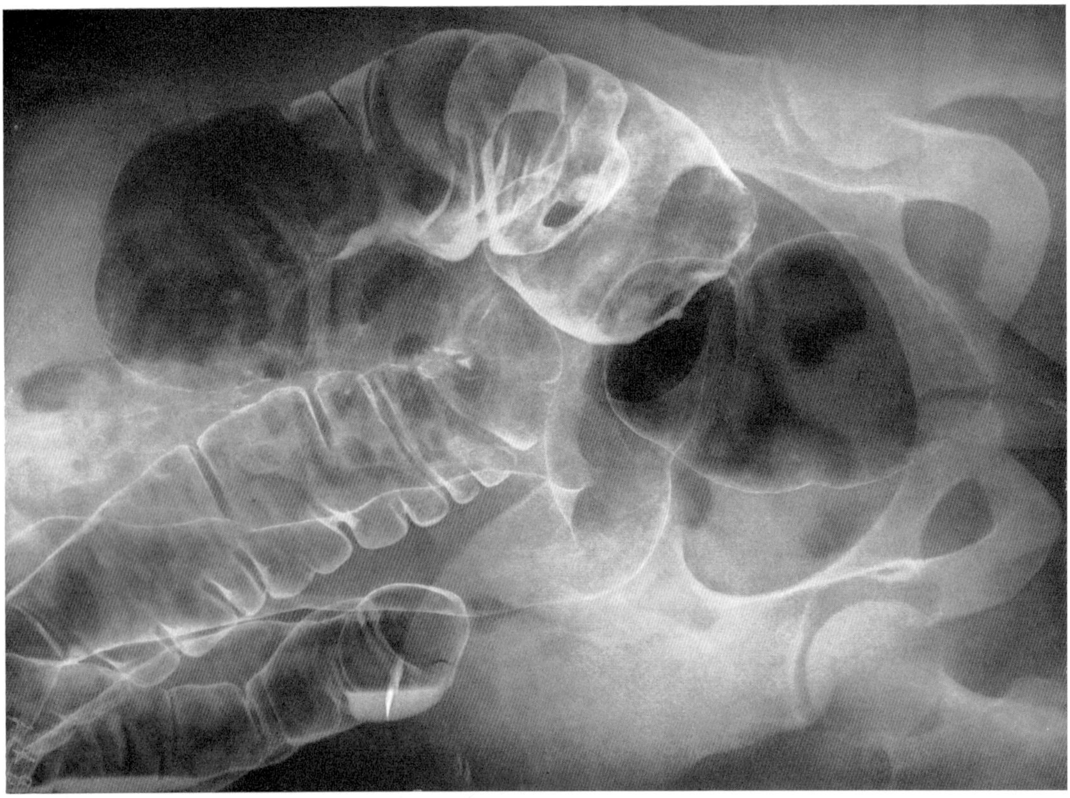

Fig. 8 Standard projection, Left recumbent position with horizontal beam.

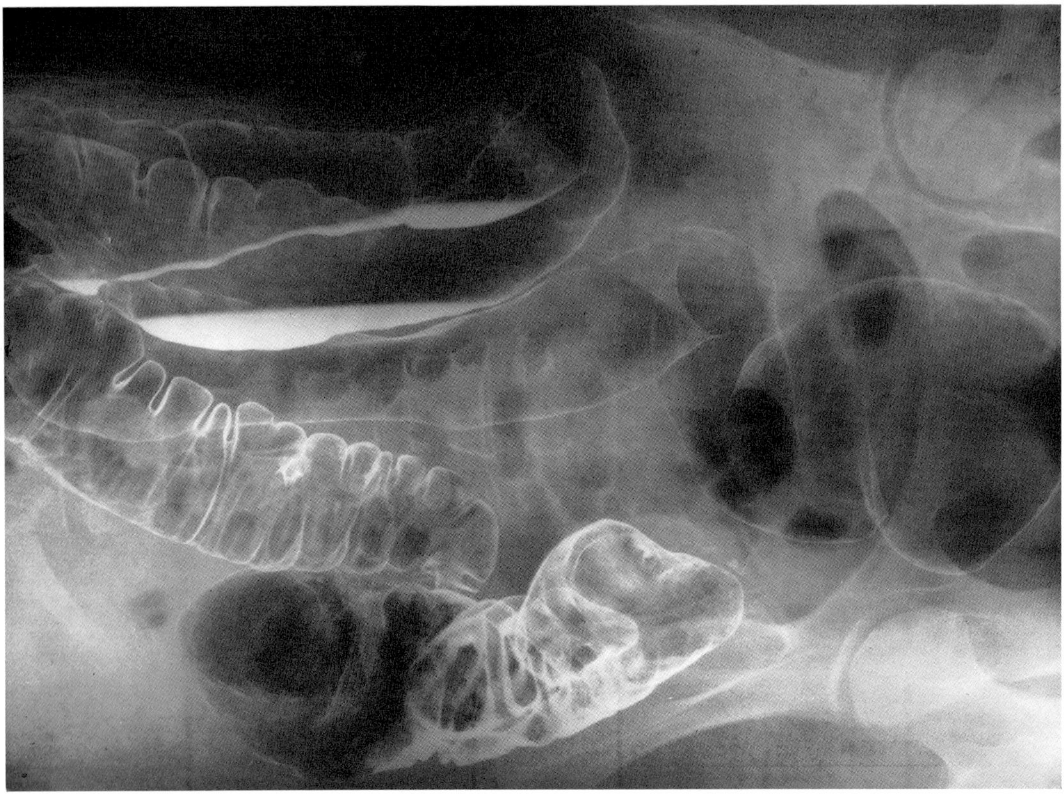

Fig. 9 Standard projection. Right recumbent position with horizontal beam.

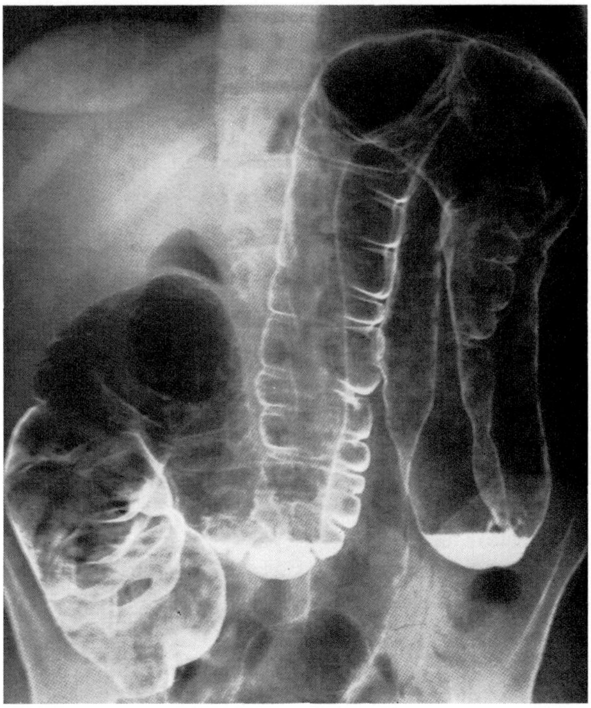

Fig. 10 Standard projection. Frontal view. Patient standing.

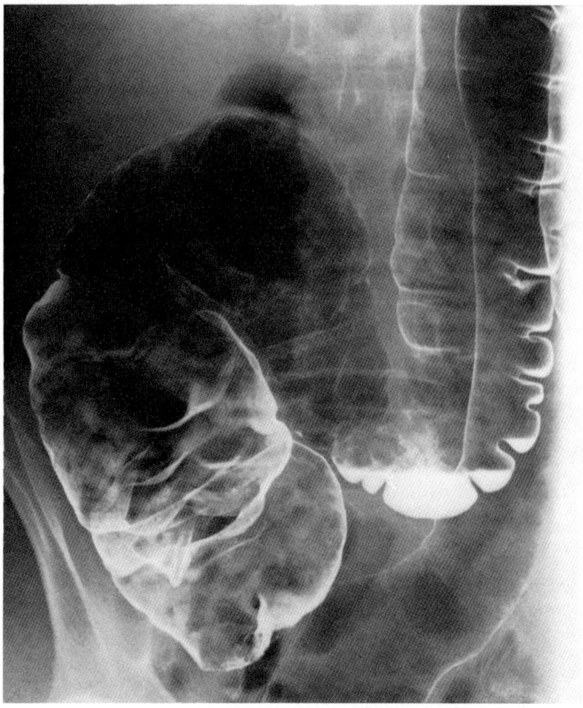

Fig. 11 Standard projection. Right anterior oblique view. Patient standing.

3. Two roentgenograms of the abdomen, especially of the hepatic flexure and splenic flexure with the patient supine and turned 30–45° to the left and to the right, respectively. Film size 30 × 40 cm. Figs. 6 and 7.
4. Roentgenograms with the patient in the right and left lateral position with the roentgen beam horizontal and with the grid respectively in front of and behind the patient. Film size 30 × 40 cm. Figs. 8 and 9.
5. Roentgenograms with the patient standing and with the beam horizontal, a frontal view and two oblique lateral views so that the hepatic flexure and splenic flexure are projected free. Film size 30 × 40 and 24 × 30 cm. Figs. 10, 11 and 12.

As previously mentioned, such a set of roentgenograms permits a very good examination of every single segment of the intestinal wall. The choice of projections depends on the variations, the size, position and form of the individual colon and enables a three-dimensional examination of the organ to be made.

When deciding upon this schedule, the difficulties of a perfect emptying of the colon were taken into consideration. Residual contrast medium

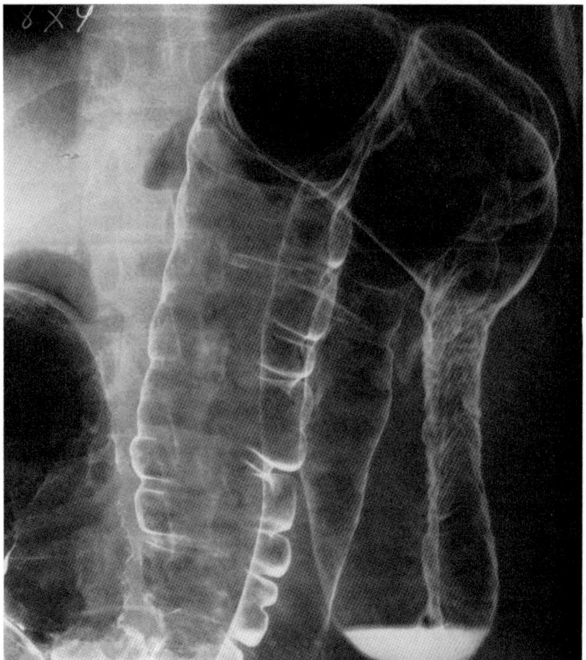

Fig. 12 Standard projection. Left anterior oblique view. Patient standing.

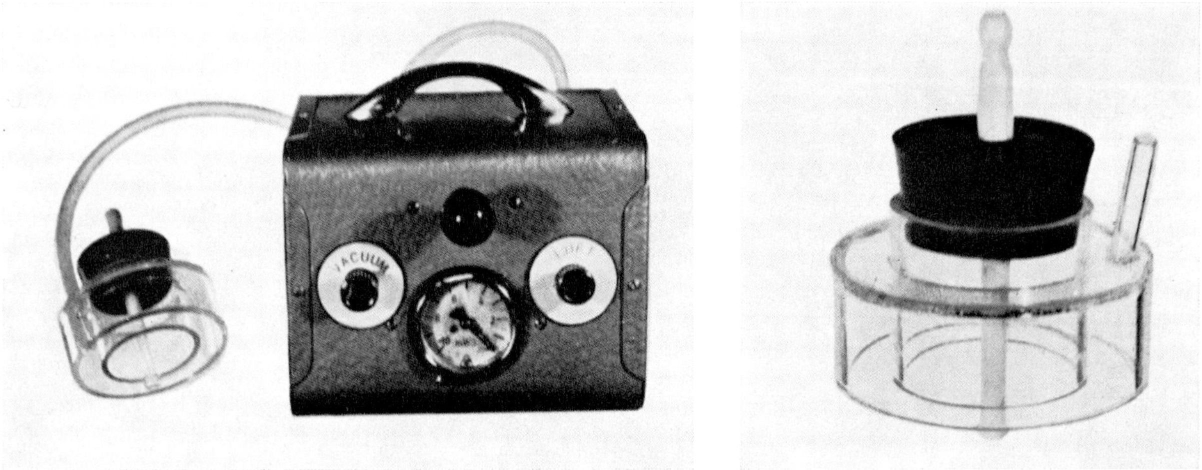

Fig. 13 Almén's instrument for examination of patients with colostomy:
a) The device
b) The Perspex cup: pipe for infusion of contrast medium inserted through rubber plug into the cylinder.

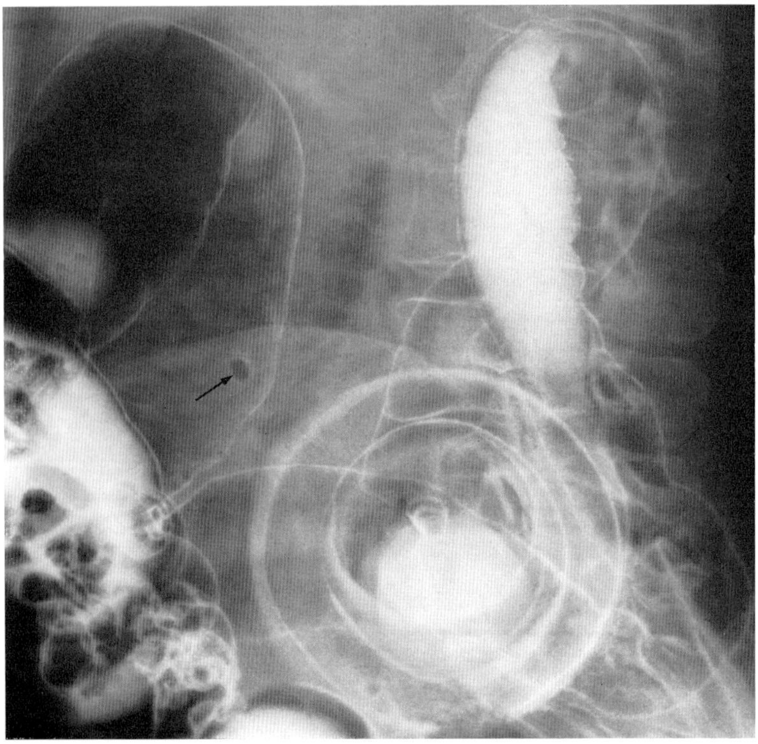

Fig. 14 ♂ 81 years. X-ray 29/8/63. Double contrast roentgenograph of a colostomized patient with Almén's device in posititon. Sentinel polyp, 5 × 7 mm.

accumulates in the deeper parts of the intestine and can then mask small lesions, but by examining the patient in the left and right lateral positions as well as standing with the beam horizontal, all segments of the intestine can be examined. The roentgenograms taken with the beam horizontal have proved very valuable.
For the examination of patients with a colostomy, we use a special device designed by Almén (1965). It is a double plastic ring, in which a partial vacuum or suction can be applied to the outer compartment. This provides an airtight seal. The seal then holds the instrument to the patient and prevents spilling of the contrast medium on to the patient and the table (Fig. 13).
The contrast medium, both barium and air, can be infused through the center of this device; with this instrument it is easy to obtain double contrast films even in a colostomized patient (Fig. 14).

5 Complications

Perforation of the large intestine during roentgen examination with the double contrast method is extremely rare. In the Malmö material, about 60,000 examinations, perforation due to increased intraintestinal pressure has never occurred. But in 2 cases the intestinal wall was perforated owing to instrumental injury. In one case sigmoidoscopy revealed the site of the perforation which had most likely been caused by the rectal tube. In the other case the patient was not examined sigmoidoscopically after the roentgen examination, but the roentgenographic appearance of the escape of air suggested a similar cause of the injury. Since the rubber rectal tubes used at that time become rigid from repeated sterilization by steam and pressure, we discarded all tubes as soon as any such rigidity was noticed. It is noteworthy that no barium had escaped in either of these cases. It may therefore be assumed that the perforation was small and closed spontaneously on relief of the increased intraintestinal pressure.

6 Polyps

Introduction

The word polyp designates any congenital or acquired neoplasm of the mucosa. The etiology of these lesions is still obscure and no effective prophylaxis is available. The importance of an early diagnosis has been the subject of much discussion, especially since pathologists claimed in the early 1950's that carcinoma of the colon and rectum often developed from such polypoid lesions. This postulation placed higher demands on the roentgenologic diagnosis. It was necessary to refine the technique so that it could demonstrate changes down to a few millimeters in diameter.

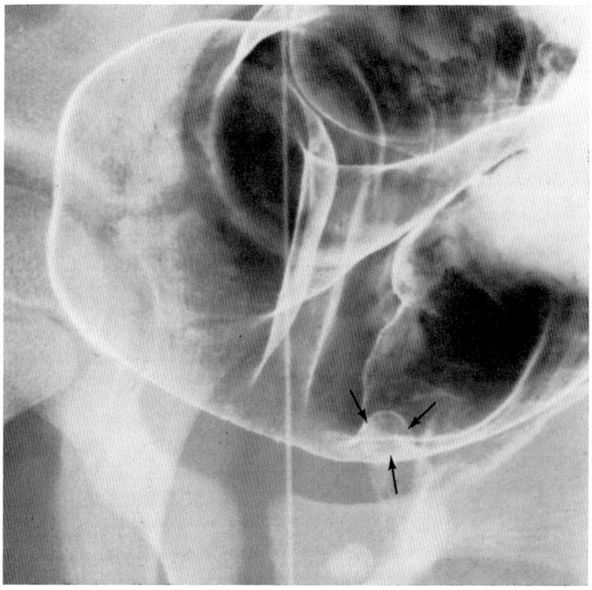

Fig. 15 ♀ 7 years. X-ray 7/4/55. Sessile polyp, measuring 4×7 mm.

Different Types of Polyps

Formerly, two morphologic types of polyps were recognized, sessile and pedunculated, but with this new modification of the double contrast examination it has been possible to distinguish a third type, which is called the intermediate or protuberant type. All three types have their own roentgenographic characteristics and can be differentiated by the appearance of the base. This is most important. The base is continuous with part of the actual mucosa and its appearance usually indicates the nature of the polyp. The profile of the sessile polyp may bulge distinctly into the lumen of the colon or it may be extremely flat.

Fig. 15 shows that the intestine is insufflated. The intestine is clean. The profile of the intestinal wall depicts the even thin film of contrast medium and the typical outline of a sessile polyp. The polyp protrudes like a stud into the lumen. It is 4 by 7 mm.

The largest polyp in Fig. 16 is flatter and in this case it is necessary to be on the lookout for an

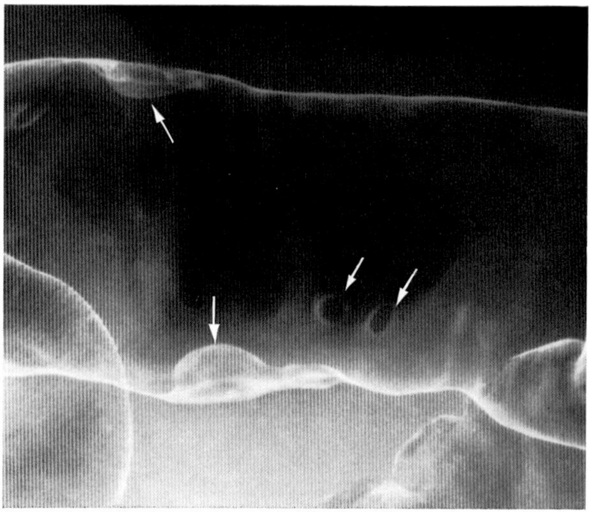

Fig. 16 ♀ 13 years. X-ray 7/4/55. 4 polyps. The largest flat, broad-based, measuring 5×11 mm.

indentation, which is a sign of malignant infiltration. (See below, p. 31.)
In facial views (Fig. 17) these polyps appear more or less rounded, and produce the picture of a ring of barium.
The sessile polyp may be a slowly growing, benign, non-infiltrating adenomatous polyp, or a rapidly infiltrating malignant tumor invading the deeper layers of the bowel. When the tumors are small, it is not possible to decide whether they are malignant or not.
Most pedunculated polyps are situated in the descending colon and the sigmoid. The development of the pedicle is caused, according to Castleman, by the fact that adenomas are usually small and do not grow invasively. The plaques can therefore be lifted up by traction of the fecal stream and by the peristaltic waves, until their base is drawn out into a stalk.
The pedicle of the polyp may be identified in profile either by its thin coating of barium surrounded by air, or as a negative shadow in an area of residual barium.
Fig. 18 illustrates a large pedunculated polyp with an irregular surface, a large pedicle in the descending colon and a small one in the splenic flexure. Both can be diagnosed from the thin coating of barium surrounded by air.
If there is superfluous barium in the intestine, the pedicle and the polyp may appear as a negative shadow (Fig. 19).
If the central ray of the roentgen beam passes parallel to the long axis of the pedicle, the barium coated pedicle will appear as a small white circle within the larger circle of barium covering the body of the polyp. In other words, it will resemble a bull's eye or a target (Fig. 20).
The pedunculated polyps usually offer no diagnostic difficulty, but so far it has not been possible to decide from their roentgenographic appearance whether they are benign or malignant.

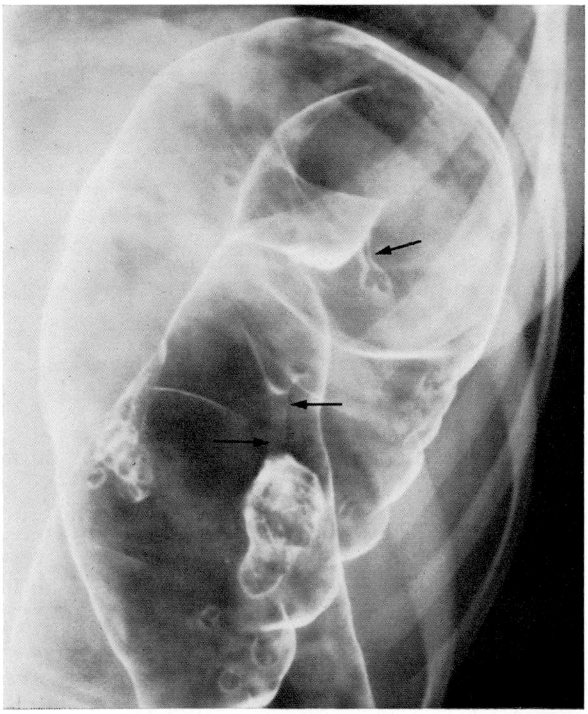

Fig. 18 ♀ 17 years. X-ray 30/4/58. Two pedunculated polyps in profile.

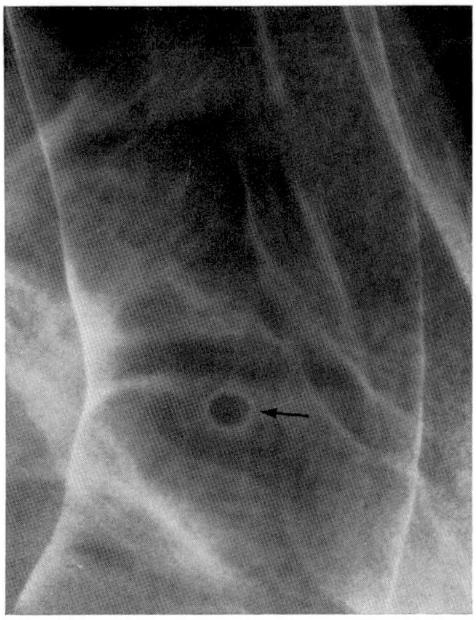

Fig. 17 ♂ 54 years. X-ray 15/11/58. Axial view of a sessile polyp, 4 mm in diameter.

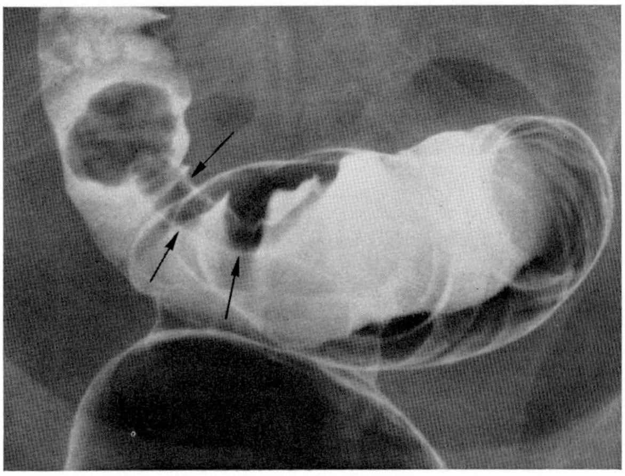

Fig. 19 ♂ 71 years. X-ray 13/3/58. Pedunculated polyp as a negative.

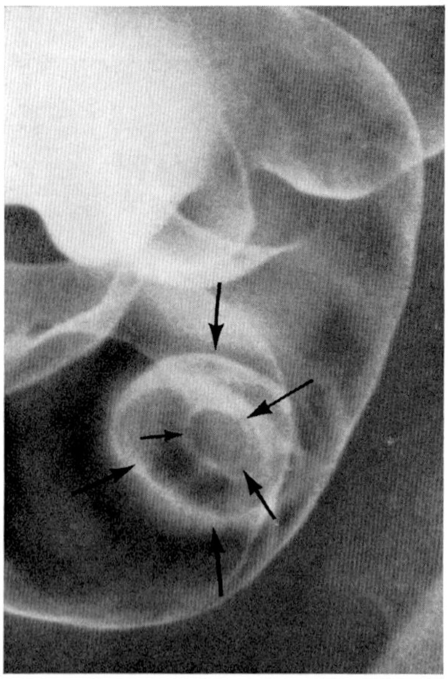

Fig. 20 ♀ 73 years. X-ray 17/5/55. Axial view of a pedunculated polyp. "Target phenomenon".

Occasionally a polyp with a stalk may be misdiagnosed as a broad-based or intermediate tumor.

In the third type, the intermediate or protuberant polyp, the adenomatous tissue is heaped into a protuberant mass with its broad base resting on the bowel wall. The appearance leaves the impression that the traction has not existed long enough to produce a stalk.

At first, the well known American pathologist Ackerman, who is particularly interested in this field, was doubtful as to this new type of polypoid formation, as he had not observed any such lesion in his pathologic examinations. However, at histologic examination of roentgenologically demonstrated protuberant polyps, he found a central fibrous core in the microscopic sections. Ackerman thought that the core was a potential stalk.

In this type of polyp there is a small recess between the base of the polyp and the bowel wall. This recess is filled with barium at the air contrast enema examination. Barium will also coat the body of the polyp and hence two white rings will appear. The relationship between these two rings is determined by the angle at which the roentgen ray beam meets the barium-coated broad-based polyp.

In an oblique view of this polyp, the thinner barium covering the polypoid body will be overlapped by the denser white ring of barium in the recess around the base (Fig. 21a). This is pathognomonic and it may be likened to a bowler hat, where the barium coated body of the polyp represents the crown and the barium around the base the brim.

In facial views of this polyp (Fig. 21b) there will be a single circle, because the ring of barium over the polyp and the ring around the base overlap.

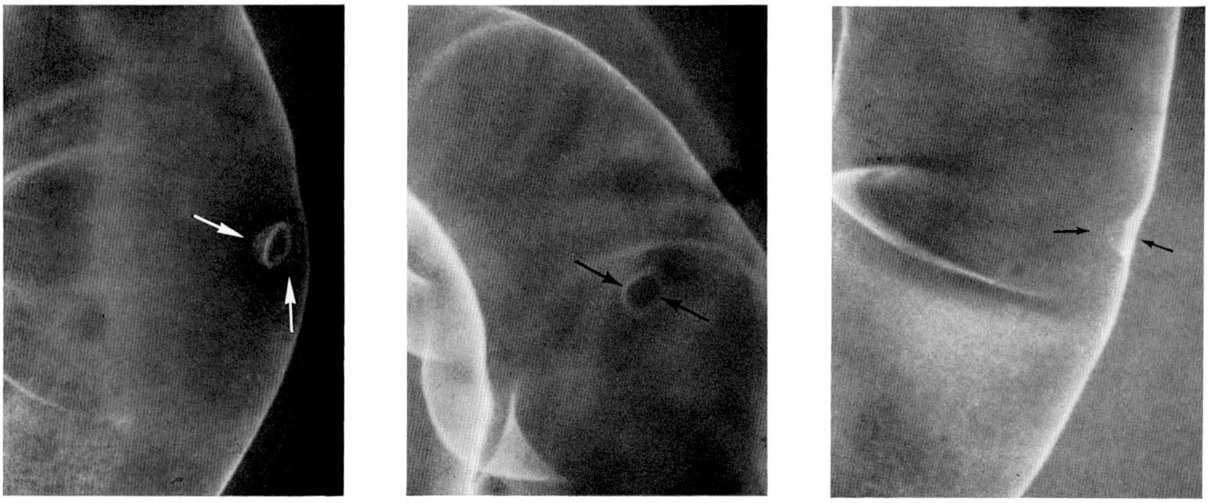

a b c

Fig. 21 ♂ 65 years. X-ray 19/3/55. Intermediate polyp:

a) Oblique view of the polyp, 3×5 mm. Two rings, the thinner one caused by the barium covering the polypoid body; the denser by barium in recess around base.

b) Axial view of the same polyp.

c) Profile view of the same polyp.

In profile the lesion (Fig. 21c) will leave the impression of an ordinary sessile polyp.
Some polypoid tumors of this type are very small. The material of this third type is not yet large enough to allow any conclusions as to whether they are potentially malignant.

Frequency of Polyps

The frequency with which polyps has been demonstrated varies from series to series. Table 2 summarizes the frequencies of polyps found in various postmortem series.

Table 2. Incidence of Polyps in Various Postmortem Series

Author	Year	No. examined	% Incidence
Lawrence	1936	7,000	2.37
Stewart	1931	1,815	4.19
Susman	1932	1,100	6.0
Lingdren	1956	1,351	7.4
Helwig	1947	1,460	9.5
Winblad and Frieberg	1956	676	11.0
De Stefano and Horwarth	1959	496	11.3
Ekelund	1963	3,398	12.50
Jackman	1941	2,874	12.60
Smedal	1941	827	14.5
Swinton and Haugh	1947	1,843	17.63
Feyrter	1931	1,800	21.4
Blatt*	1961	446	38.8

* Patients over 30 years old

The frequency also varies considerably in the clinical series. This can probably be ascribed, at least partly, to differences in the composition of the series studied. Some series consisted of routine examinations; others, of patients with colonic symptoms. In addition, the variation may be due partly to the fact that some of the frequencies were based only on sigmoidoscopic findings, others partly on sigmoidoscopic and partly on roentgenographic findings and the remainder on roentgenographic findings alone. The age distribution of the materials studied also plays a certain role because the frequency of polyps is known to be higher in the higher age groups.
At sigmoidoscopy of 1,693 patients Martin (1939) found polyps in 75 and carcinoma in 50 cases. Green (1941) found polyps in 10.8 percent of 640 patients, Ortmayer (1950) in 3 percent of 3,450 women, Binkley (1952) in 6.4 percent of 300 patients and Burnikel and Schutte (1954) in 9.8 percent of 5,072 patients. Rider (1954) who examined 7,489 patients, found polyps in 401 and in a later paper on a material of 9,669 examinations in 537 (5.5 percent). Walske found polyps in 15 percent of 1,000 consecutive patients. All of his patients had been admitted to hospital for reasons other than symptoms referable to the intestine. In an analysis by Portes and Majarakis (1957) of the sigmoidoscopic findings in 50,000 patients examined at the Cancer Prevention Center the frequency of polyps was found to be 7.9 percent.
Thus, of the clinical series on record, the frequency varied between 3 and 15 percent.
Combined sigmoidoscopy and roentgen examination with the high voltage technique was used by Gianturco. In 1950 he reported that he had found polyps in 2.7 percent of 1,552 examinations. In 1957 Enquist published his experience at The Cancer Detection Center at the University of Minnesota. His material consisted of 7,608 symptom-free patients and the examinations were carried out between March 1, 1948 and February 28, 1956. Sigmoidoscopy and roentgen examination revealed one or more polyps in the rectum or colon of 1,462 (19.2 percent) patients.
Rosenzweig and Horwitz (1958) examined 777 patients with sigmoidoscopy and the double contrast method and found polyps in 188 (24.2 percent). In 59 (31.4 percent) of these patients the neoplasms were multiple.
Even in series examined by roentgenography alone, the results have varied considerably. This variation was due mainly to different techniques used. With the old barium enema it was only occasionally possible to demonstrate such small lesions. Garret (1950), for instance, stressed that barium enema is of little value for diagnosing small lesions in the rectum. According to Weber, polypoid formations 2 cm or less in diameter will nearly always escape even meticulous examination and leave the examiner in doubt about the reliability of his diagnosis.
Finney and Stone (1953) wrote that it must be realized that the barium enema is not really reliable and does not always give the correct diagnosis, no matter how thoroughly and technically the examination is performed or how skilfully the interpretation may be made.

With the so-called mucosal relief technique small lesions down to 10 mm in diameter have occasionally been demonstrated. In 1950 Christie et al. reported finding polypoid neoplasms at 40 of 4,226 examinations.

Using Gianturco's high voltage technique with diluted barium enema Wietersen (1957) found polypoid neoplasms in 31 of 1,000 consecutive examinations; of these, 24 percent were malignant. Fiegel and Fiegel (1958), who used the same method and a compression pad, demonstrated polyps in 8 percent.

With our modification of the double contrast method polypoid growths were diagnosed in 12.5 percent. The reason for this high percentage was that this modification of the double contrast method demonstrates even very small polyps. It should be stressed that these percentages were in full agreement with those found by the pathologists at Malmö hospital in two different investigations with special reference to polypoid neoplasms of the colon. In 1956 Winblad and Frieberg found polyps in 11 percent of 496 autopsy cases, and Ekelund (1958–1961) found polyps in 12.5 percent of 3,398 autopsies. This strongly suggests that our modification will demonstrate practically all polypoid tumors, even small ones, with almost the same reliability as the pathologists.

The patients in Malmö came from all departments of the hospital as well as from practitioners in the city. Most cases were examined because of symptoms suggesting disease of the colon, some for a possibly primary tumor and occasionally because of cancerophobia. The composition and age distribution of the material in Malmö was that of an ordinary hospital series.

Age Distribution

Table 3. Age Distribution of Polyps (Malmö Series)

Age	Male	Female
0–9	22.5%	16.9%
10–19	11.6	7.8
20–29	9.4	6.2
30–39	9.1	7.3
40–49	11.4	8.7
50–59	14.1	12.8
60–69	21.0	13.3
70–79	19.2	15.0
80–89	17.0	12.4

It is clear from the table that the frequency increases with age, which is in good agreement with earlier experience, though in our material it did not reach the frequency of 15 percent given by Robertson (1934) in patients aged over 50. The high percentage in childhood can probably be explained by the assumption that only those children with well-founded suspicion of intestinal polyps were examined. The frequency given is thus not the true frequency in these age classes, which is probably much lower. In the other age groups, however, there were many cases in which there was little or no reason to suspect polyp.

Polypoid neoplasms may be solitary or multiple. According to Wietersen (1957), at least 20 percent of all polyps are multiple, while Thompson and Pinck (1956) give a figure of at least 25 percent. Turell et al. (1959) gave 30 percent, Rosenzweig and Horwitz (1958) 31 percent, de Muth (1952) 33 percent, Scarborough et al. (1965) 36 percent and McMillan and Potter (1952) 40 percent. De Stefano and Horwath (1959) found one polyp in 80 percent of their patients with polyps, two in 14 percent and three or more in 6 percent. In the Malmö series the corresponding figures were 76, 17 and 7 percent.

Coexisting polyps are so common in carcinoma that they have been called "sentinel polyps". Jackman and Mayo (1958) found "sentinel polyps" in 18 percent, Leblanc (1953) in 20 percent, McMillan (1952) in 25 percent, Schmieden and Westhues (1927) in 43 percent and Dukes (1958) in 75 percent of their series of operated colonic carcinomas. In Helwig's material one or more polyps were found in more than half of all cases of carcinomas. In a group of 21 patients with multiple carcinoma Ravdin (1960) found adenoma in 50 percent. In Malmö surgeons and pathologists found polyps in 20 percent of 960 cases of operated carcinoma. Sometimes the "sentinel polyps" are remote from the site of the large tumor. It is important that the surgeon be informed of these small changes and that the sites of these be demonstrated to the surgeon, because they are often malignant.

Size of Polyps

Polyps vary widely in size. They may reach a diameter of up to 5 cm and sometimes, though rarely, the sessile polyp assumes a distinct form, known as the giant adenomatous polyp, with a diameter that may exceed 10 cm.

To appraise the frequency of polyps of various sizes we checked the roentgenograms of patients with polyps that had been operated upon and examined histologically between the 1st December 1953 and the 31 st May 1967. There were 1,134 polyps. The results are given in Table 4.

Table 4. Frequency of Polyps of Various Sizes.

Size	Number	%
0– 5 mm	424	37.4
5–10	321	28.3
10–15	157	13.8
15–20	94	8.3
20–25	48	4.2
25–30	43	3.8
30–35	17	1.5
< 35	30	2.7

As in other materials, the frequency decreased with increasing size of the polyps. 37 percent were less than 5 mm in diameter, and 65 percent less than 10 mm, while only 4 percent were more than 30 mm.

Site of Polyps

Opinions differ on the site of polyps in the colon. Most workers believe that some two-thirds of all polyps are situated within the reach of the sigmoidoscope. Table 5 shows the results of such investigations. Some authors have, however,

Table 5. Percentages of Polyps within Sigmoidoscopic Level in Published Series.

	%
Rosenzweig and Horwitz (1958)	93.4
Turell (1955)	90
Buie (1949)	85
Klein and Scarborough (1952)	81
Grinnel and Lane (1958)	79.2
Marin (1940)	77
De Stefano and Horwitz (1958)	74
Jackman and Mayo (1951)	70
Blanc and Krause (1953)	70
Sawyer (1940)	70
Stevenson and Wilson (1954)	70
Swinton and Warren (1939)	70
Smedal (1941)	68
Van Buskirk (1955)	67
Welin (1968)	67
Boehme and Hansson (1946)	65
Fitts (1954)	65
Lindgren (1956)	52

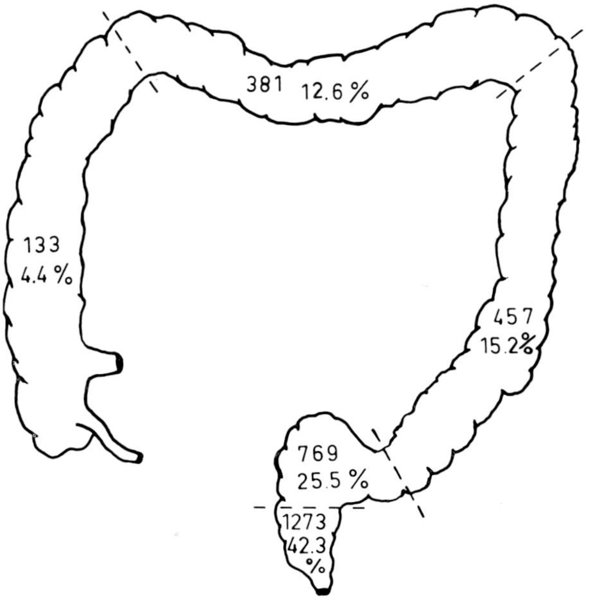

Fig. 22 Statistical distribution of polyps of the large bowel in the Malmö study.

found a different distribution. Hultborn (1952), for example, found quite a different distribution of 71 cases at autopsy. Only 16 percent of the polyps were situated in the rectum and only 19 percent in the rectosigmoid. Also Blatt (1961), who had autopsied 446 subjects personally over 30 years, diagnosed 465 polyps. He found only 7 percent in the rectum and 20 percent in the sigmoid. According to a personal communication by Fiegel in Detroit, a pathologist working in the same hospital had found similar figures. In a personal consecutive series Chapman (1963) found a change in distribution of the adenomatous polyps between the age groups 50–60 years, 60–70 years and 70–80 years. In the first-mentioned group he found 43.4 percent of the polyps in the sigmoid, compared with only 15.6 and 18 percent respectively in the second and third. The distribution of the polyps in the Malmö series examined with the double contrast method is given in Fig. 22.

Differential Roentgen Diagnosis

Pedunculated polyps have a very characteristic appearance and generally offer no diagnostic difficulties. The stalk is pathognomonic; but their differential diagnosis is often very difficult.

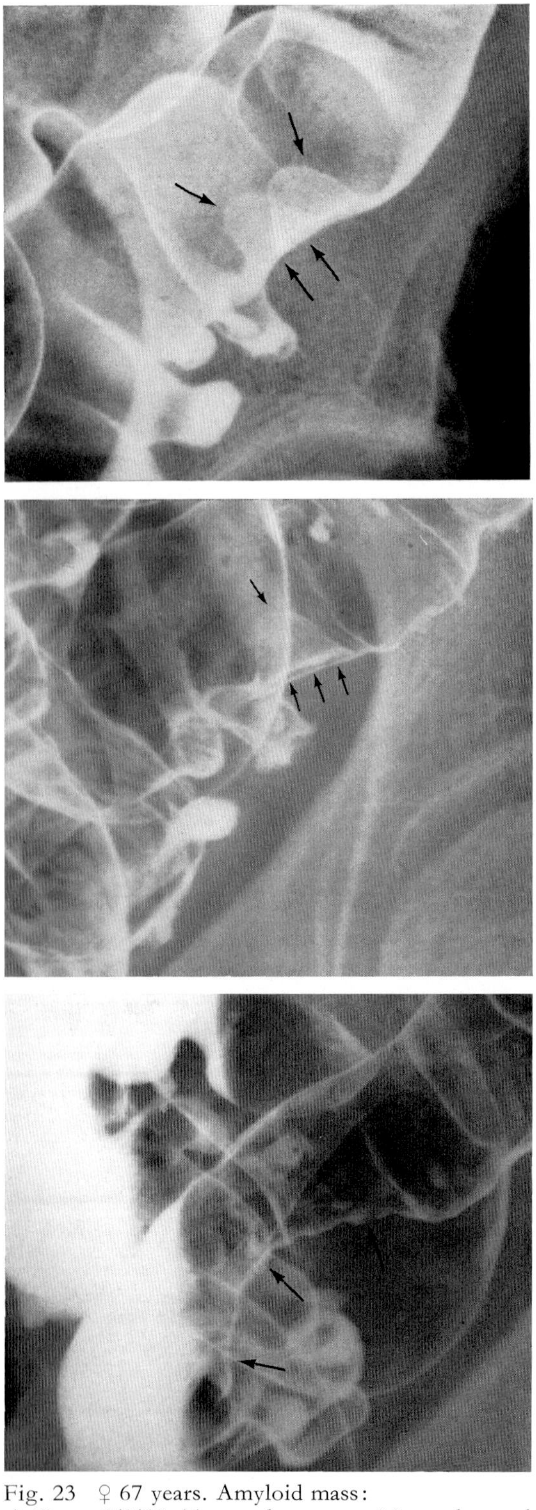

a

b

c

Fig. 23 ♀ 67 years. Amyloid mass:
a) X-ray 3/3/58. Two polyps on a 3.5 cm long plaque, causing indentation of large bowel.
b) X-ray 8/5/59. Only one polyp is now seen. The plaque is more pronounced.
c) X-ray 31/5/60. The plaque is now even larger and more rigid.

It is not possible to decide, for example, whether they are malignant or whether they are adenomatous polyps or villous papillomas.

The broad-based adenomatous polyps may sometimes offer differential diagnostic difficulties and it is generally impossible to distinguish them from benign tumors. Other lesions, such as amyloid tumors, can also exhibit similar roentgenographic changes (Fig. 23). In the reproduction (Fig. 23a) of a roentgenogram of a 67-year-old woman, examined on March 3, 1958, there are two polypoid lesions on a 3.5 cm long arcuate plaque in the intestinal wall with a strikingly even and apparently normal relief. It resembles a submucosal lesion of the wall. In the roentgenogram made on May 8, 1959 (Fig. 23b), the pathologic findings in the wall were unchanged, but only one polyp was demonstrable. In the roentgenogram of May 31, 1960 (Fig. 23c), the inwardly convex arcuate process was still more pronounced. It decreased the lumen of the intestine to about half, and the mucosa, which covered the process, appeared to be normal, though somewhat uneven. Distally in the changed area there appeared to be two small polyps. As it was not possible to exclude cancer, surgical exploration was recommended. The surgeons found the two polypoid lesions and one of them appeared to have spread in the wall. But there was no gross penetration on the serosal side. The histologic examination showed an amyloid tumor covered by a normal intestinal mucosa.

Fecal material can often cause defects liable to be confused with polypoid tumors. In most cases, however, the irregular shape, the coating and the mobility exclude polypoid lesions. In some cases, however, the fecal mass is of such an appearance that differential diagnosis is not possible, especially if the mass is so adherent to the intestinal wall that it does not change in shape or position with the posture of the body during examination. One examination in the right and left lateral position with the beam horizontal will usually clear up the diagnosis (Fig. 24). But should there still be doubt after examination with the patient in these positions, the examination must be repeated.

From time to time air bubbles cause confusion in the interpretation of the roentgenogram (Fig. 25). A thin bubble is generally surrounded by a gradually fading margin of barium. Large multiple air bubbles surrounded by many small ones are common. Such an appearance and failure to

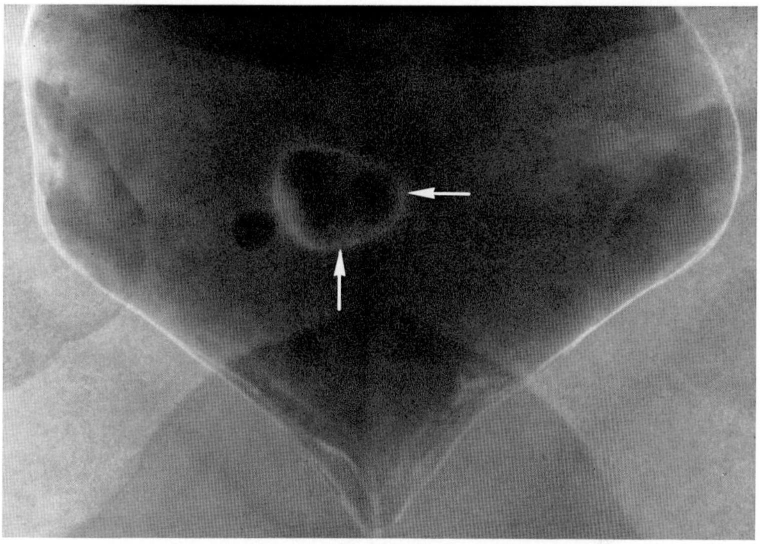

Fig. 24 ♀ 56 years. X-ray 16/2/74. Fecal material simulating a polyp:
a) Frontal view of the "suspect" polyp, 17 mm in diameter.

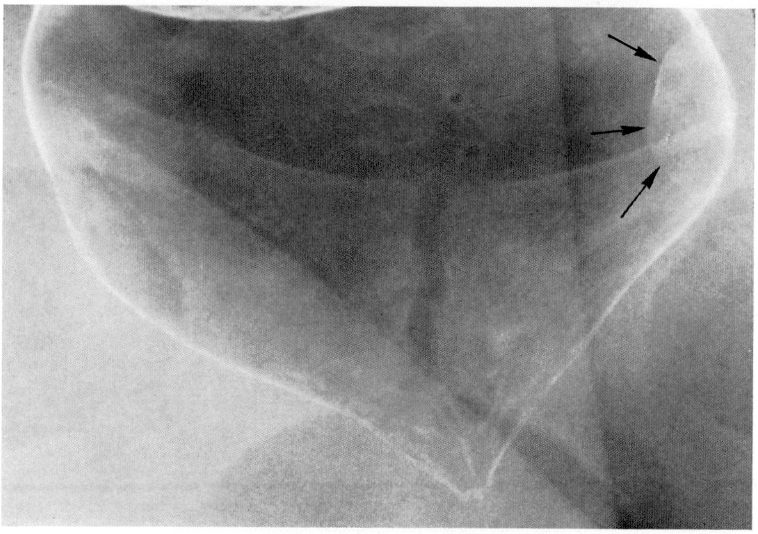

Fig. 24 b) In left recumbent position the "polyp" has moved to the left wall of the rectum.

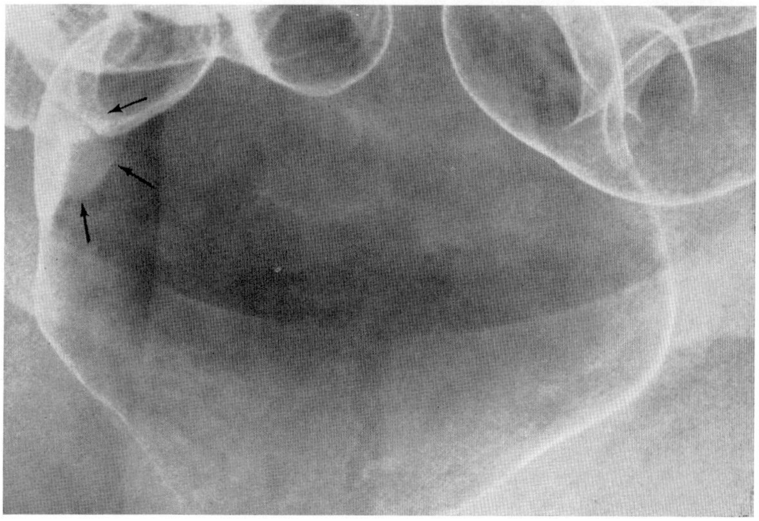

Fig. 24 c) In right recumbent position it moved to the right lateral wall.

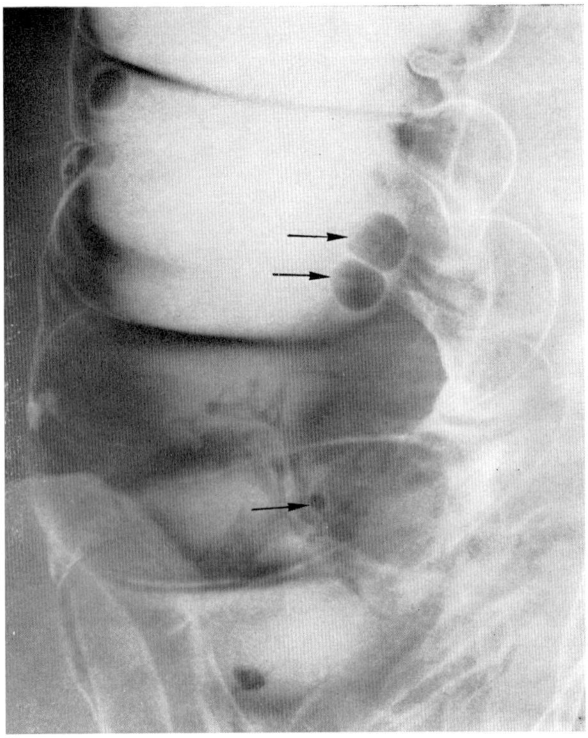

Fig. 25 ♀ 31 years. X-ray 5/11/64. Air bubbles simulating polyps.

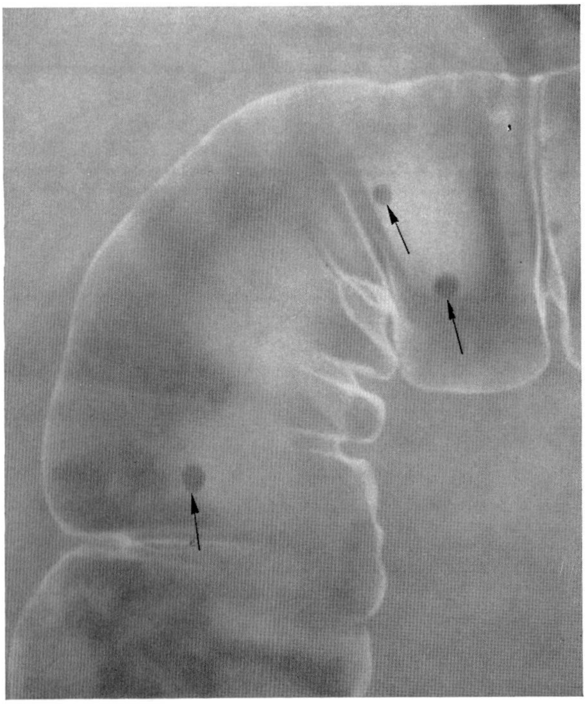

Fig. 26 ♂ 57 years. X-ray 21/12/61. Oil droplets simulating polyps.

demonstrate the base exclude a real polypoid lesion.

Oil bubbles due to excessive castor oil are similar in appearance (Fig. 26). Fat should not be applied to the intestine or the enema tube. But, owing to their instability and radiolucency and their usually thick, homogenous and very well defined outline, oil bubbles are easy to distinguish from neoplasms.

Occasionally strands of mucus produce long slender defects within the barium. Owing to the changing widths of these strands they are easily identified. These problems are now excluded by the use of atropine.

Barium-coated diverticula protruding beyond the bowel wall do not offer any differential diagnostic difficulty. In frontal views they resemble polyps; but even then it is possible to make a differential diagnosis (Fig. 27). The roentgenological appearance of a diverticulum is characterized by a ring of barium with a sharp outer border and a diffuse inner contour. On the other hand, the barium coating of a polyp is sharp on its inner, and poorly defined on its outer, border. The difference is because barium is inside the diverticulum, but outside the polyp.

Calcified blood vessels (Fig. 28 a, b), lymph nodes, genital calcifications and sclerotic skeletal changes (Fig. 29 a, b) can also sometimes be

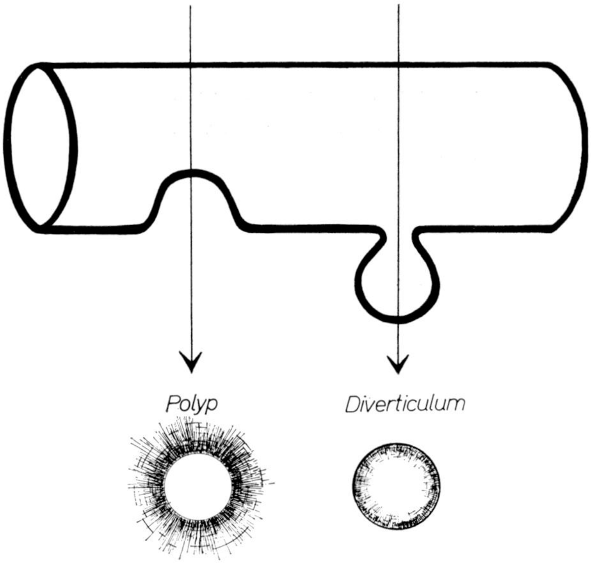

Fig. 27 Schematic demonstration of difference between polyp and diverticulum in the roentgenogram. In axial view the polyp has a sharp inner and indistinct outer margin. The diverticulum presents a reversal of these findings.

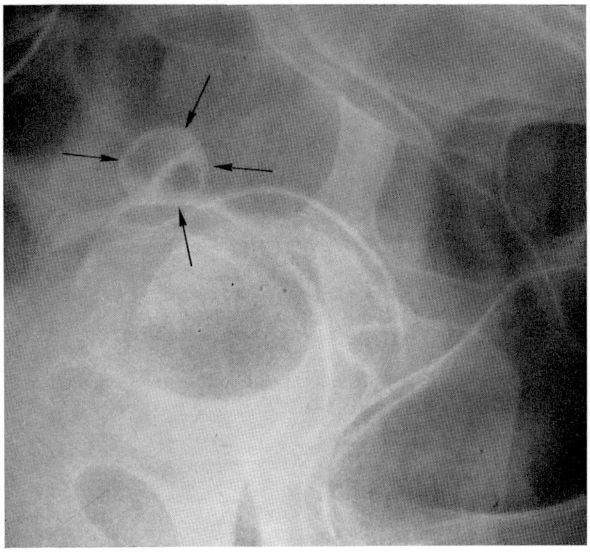

a

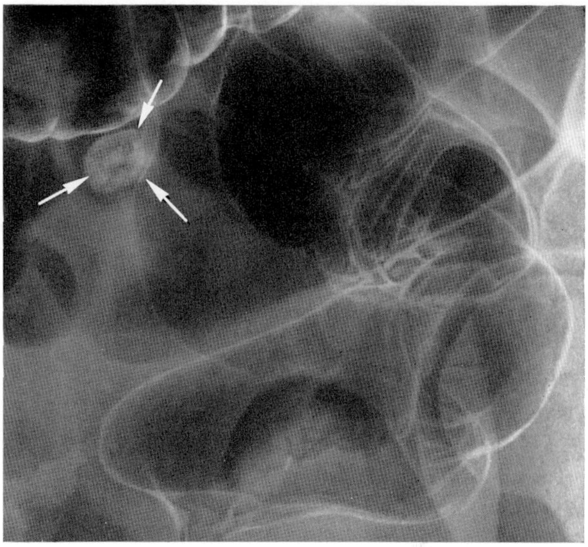

b

Fig. 28 ♀ 50 years. X-ray 25/1/60. a), b) Calcification in a vessel, simulating a polyp.

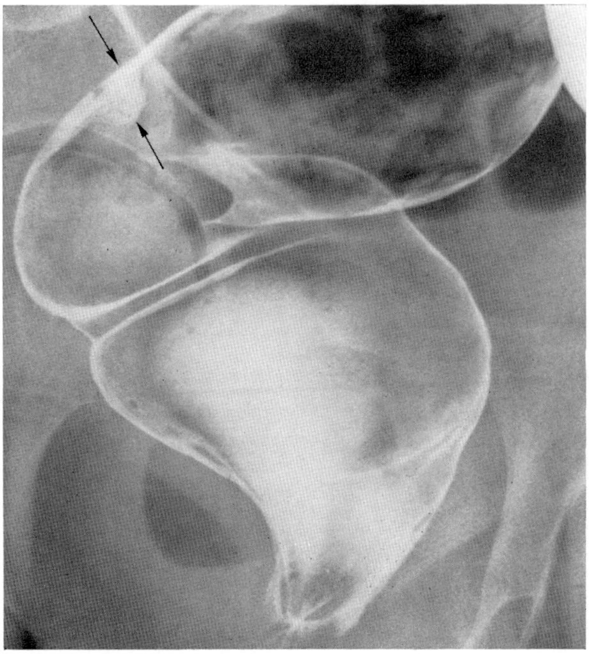

a

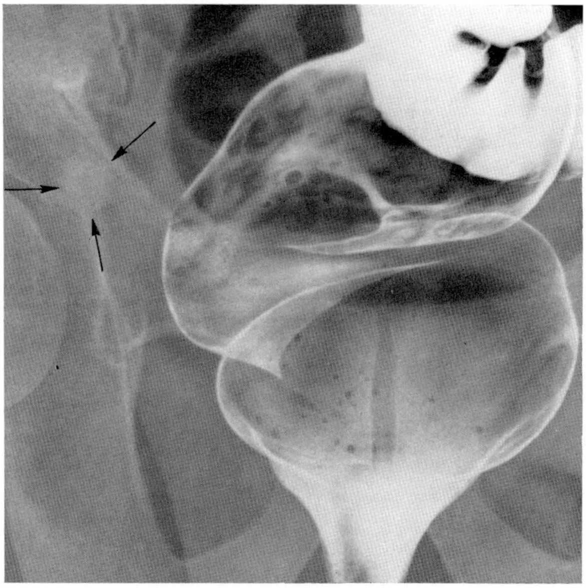

b

Fig. 29 ♂ 54 years. X-ray 12/12/61. a), b) Sclerotic plaque in pelvis simulating a polyp.

mistaken for polyps, but the change in their position relative to the intestine in different projections usually makes a differential diagnosis possible.

Granuloma (Fig. 30) and folds in the intestine (Fig. 31) can also sometimes cause differential diagnostic difficulties, as can an enlarged valvula Bauhini (Figs. 32 a, b).

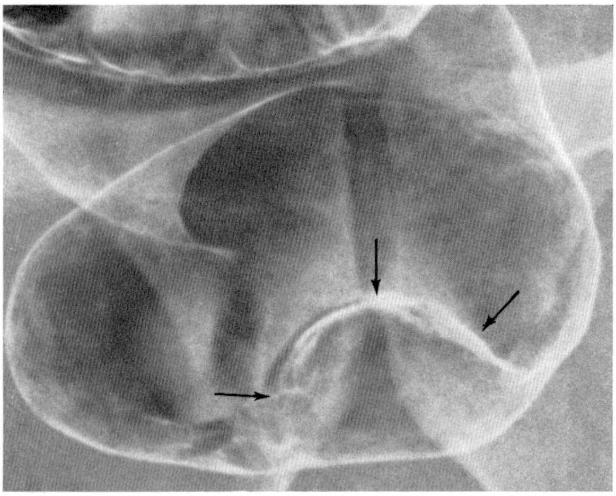

Fig. 30 ♂ 54 years. X-ray 29/10/57. Phenol granuloma simulating a polyp.

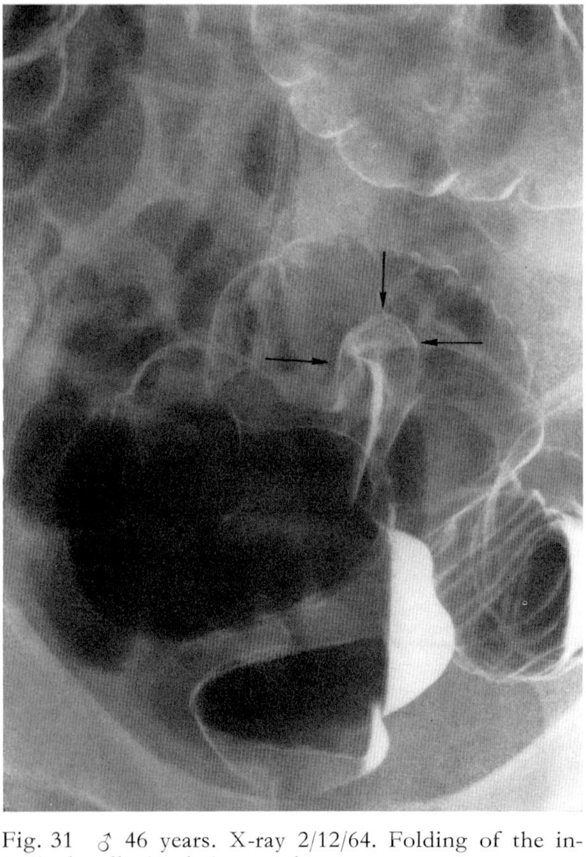

Fig. 31 ♂ 46 years. X-ray 2/12/64. Folding of the intestinal wall, simulating a polyp.

After appendectomy the stump of the appendix may sometimes be mistaken for a polyp in the roentgenogram (Figs. 33 a, b, c), and in the region of the cecum one must bear in mind the possibility of local neoplasms, such as a mucocele or a granuloma on the appendix.

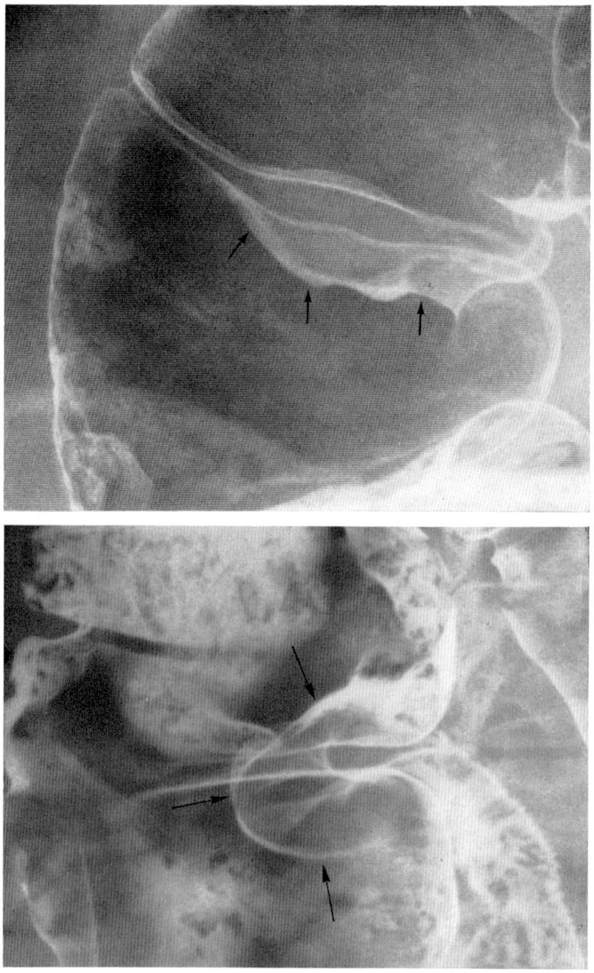

Fig. 32 ♀ 51 years. X-ray 19/9/63. a), b) Protrusion of enlarged valve of Bauhini, simulating neoplasm.

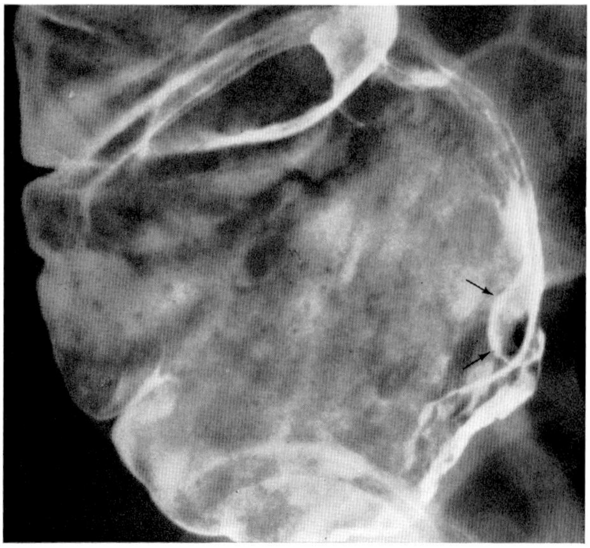

Fig. 33 a) ♀ 52 years. X-ray 24/4/56. Invagination of an appendiceal stump, simulating a polypoid tumor.

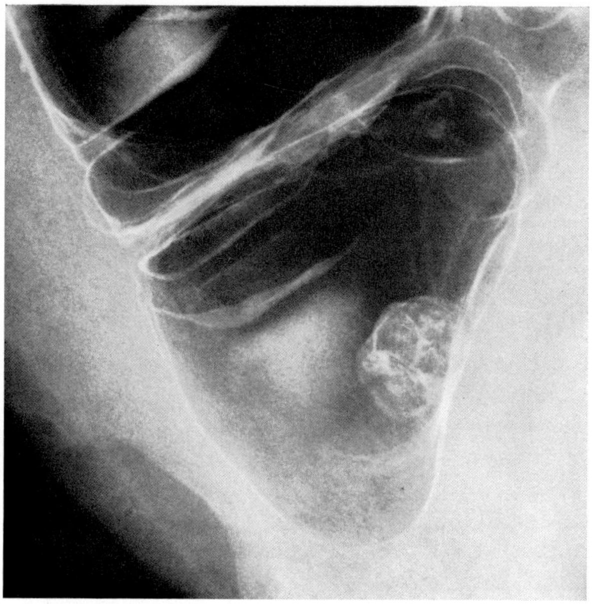

Fig. 33 b) ♀ 65 years. X-ray 17/6/54. Sessile polyp.

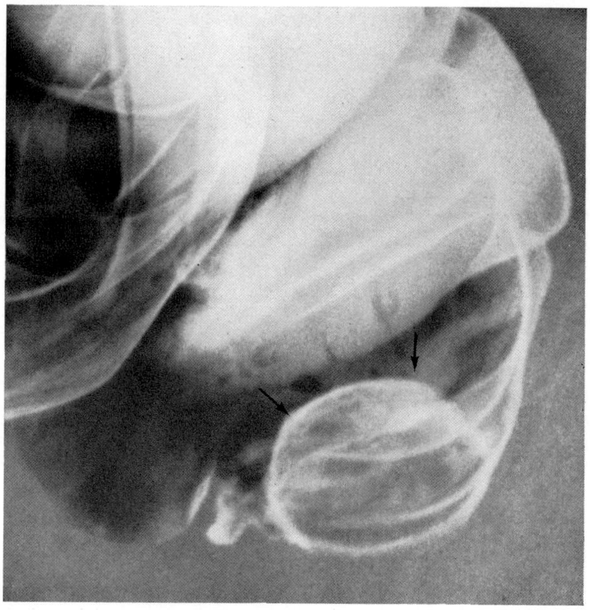

Fig. 33 c) ♂ 61 years. X-ray 19/8/60. Mucocele.

Pathology

Benign tumors of the large intestine are more common than in any other part of the digestive tract. They are most often adenomatous polyps – according to Ravdin (1960) 95 percent of all epithelial tumors of the large intestine. Adenomas have attracted much attention because many investigators claim that there must be a close connection between these small tumors and cancer. The appraisal of the relationship of adenomas of the colon to carcinomas raises many questions. The propensity of the polyp to become malignant is one of the most debated and controversial subjects in medicine. Numerous surveys have appeared in the literature and much has been written for and against the theory.

Today most pathologists are of the opinion that adenomatous polyps are either precancerous or potentially malignant. Even Versé (1908), Dukes (1925), Erdman and Morris (1925) stated that these polyps have a strong tendency to become malignant. Their opinion was based mainly on findings of small carcinomatous foci in otherwise benign polyps.

Other research workers also soon began to believe that they could histologically prove the development of a benign polyp to a malignant process. For instance, Schmieden and Westhues (1927) postulated that their material suggested that carcinoma can develop from a polypoid prestage and that 50 percent of all polyps developed into malignant growths. Also Swinton and Warren (1939) claimed to have shown histologically that more than 14 percent of their 827 cases of carcinoma of the colon and rectum had developed from benign polyps. Bockus (1961) published a survey according to which 5–85 percent of all originally benign rectal polyps had become malignant with time.

In 1931 Fitzgibbon published a paper in which he stated that he had found residual polypoid tissue in 22 of 24 carcinomas. He therefore felt it probable that the histogenesis of carcinoma of the colon developed from a precancerous polyp. Helwig (1952) demonstrated 12 cases of small carcinomas, 10 of which had their origin in an adenoma. According to Helwig, there was histologic as well as cytologic evidence that an adenoma can degenerate into a malignant growth.

Martin (1939) was of the view that the large majority of polyps of the colon and rectum, if not all, became malignant with time provided that the patient lived long enough, unless they were removed. Also Lockhart-Mummery (1934), Buie (1937), Brust (1942) and Dockerty (1958) were of the opinion that all polypous adenomas are potentially malignant and clearly tend to become malignant sooner or later. Sawyer (1940) claimed that the probability of polyps in a given patient becoming malignant depends on their number and that in disseminated polyposis it is 100 percent.

Jackman (1951), Mayo and Bacon (1951) were all convinced that adenomatous polyps can become carcinomatous and Robertson (1934), Atwater and Bargen (1945), McMillan and Potter (1952), Hultborn (1954) and many others regarded the adenoma as a stage in the development of a malignant clinical picture and considered it as a clearly precancerous condition. The only carcinomas of the rectum and colon which are not of polypoid origin are, according to Tucker (1940) the intramural mucoidal carcinoma, which develops in the intestinal wall and those carcinomas which develop in anal fistula or anal fissure.

There is also other evidence of an intimate connection between polyps and malignant tumors, namely:

1. The coexistence of benign adenoma and polypoid adenocarcinoma.
2. The development of adenocarcinoma at the site of a previously observed apparently benign adenoma.
3. The diagnosis of colonic cancer in patients 10 years older on the average than those with benign polypoid tumors.
4. The development of an adenoma during the so-called cancer age.
5. The high rate of benign polyps as well as adenocarcinomas in the rectum and sigmoid colon – Catell and Swinton (1937) suggest for example that 68 percent of all adenomas and 60 percent of all carcinomas are situated in the rectum and sigmoid.
6. In the other segments of the large intestine too there is a certain parallelism between the positions of the benign polyps and carcinomas.
7. The frequency with which the polyps are associated with carcinomas.
8. Death from carcinoma of the colon of almost all untreated patients with familial polyposis.

According to Wangensteen (1949), a polyp can become carcinomatous within 2 years, while Helwig (1947), Dedisch et al. (1955), Myers and Bacon (1960) feel that such degeneration requires several years.

These authors are thus convinced that it is a question of an originally benign neoplasm which later develops into cancer, and as early as 1948 Cattel stated that the greatest opportunity in the future for the improvement of results lies in the discovery and treatment of the premalignant lesion of the colon and rectum, the benign polyp. He also stressed that the adenocarcinoma constitutes about 99 percent of all cancers of the colon and rectum. In the early 1950s the American pathologists coined the slogan "Polyp detection is cancer prevention".

But there are still some research workers who are in doubt about the malignant degeneration of adenomatous polyps. They claim that most of the polyps are benign and remain so. They point out that in children carcinoma of the colon is rare, while polyps are fairly common. They believe that the risk of degeneration of a given polyp to cancer must be low. Ackerman and del Regato (1962) expressed the opinion that adenoma plays no essential role in the development of cancer. In his series Ackerman was unable to find any residual polyps or remains of polyps in 298 cases diagnosed by him as carcinoma. Of 425 polyps he found only one with suspect infiltration of the stem. He thought these results were incompatible with the theory that adenomatous polyps are substantially responsible for the development of malignant tumors of the colon. He felt that the adenomatous polyp of the colon might be equated with those found in Peutz-Jegher's syndrome and which are generally regarded as benign. Ackerman and Spratt (1962) thought that if the carcinoma arose in adenomas, the best chance of finding adenomatous tissue in cancer would be in small lesions. They therefore carefully sectioned 20 small cancers and found no evidence of benign tissue. David (1934) stressed that polyps are very often found which have existed for a long time and have not become malignant. He also stressed that it is by no means uncommon that polyps are diagnosed in children, in whom carcinoma of the colon is rare. Feyrter (1929) also felt that degeneration of a polypous adenoma to a carcinoma is rare. Rider (1954) claimed that he had never in his investigation found evidence of such a malignant degeneration of an originally benign neoplasm. Boyd (1951), Weingarten (1952), Ortmayer (1956) and other authors stressed that such degeneration still remains to be proved.

A third group of investigators consider malignancy to have been present from the very beginning. To this group belong Colvert and Brown

(1948). On the basis of their material they conclude that malignant tumors are malignant from the very beginning or at any rate become so very early, while benign polyps do not become malignant with time. They therefore claimed that it is difficult to establish the prognosis in a given case.
However, regardless which of these opinions is right, i.e. whether the polyps are malignant, potentially malignant or not malignant at all, an early diagnosis of these small neoplasms is of paramount importance. There is now almost general agreement that radical removal of the polyps would constitute a real prophylaxis, against carcinomas of the colon.

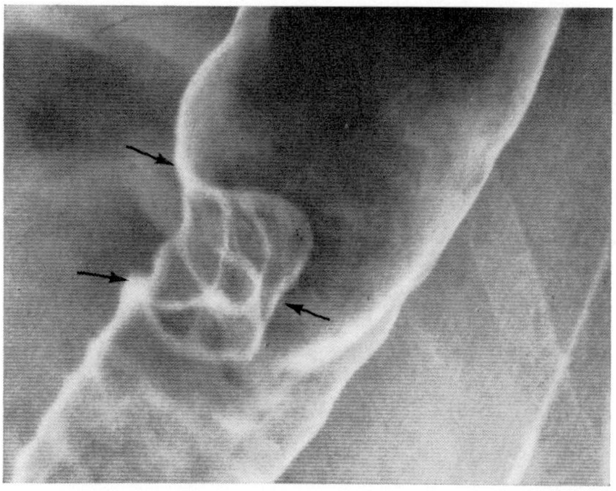

Fig. 34 a) ♀ 49 years. X-ray 12/10/55. Sessile polyp, 13 × 18 mm with typical indentation – cancer.

Roentgenographic Changes Suggesting Malignancy

Surgical removal of all these small tumors would mostly not be realistic, even if the pathologist's view that a radical removal would constitute a real prophylaxis against cancer of the colon is correct. It was therefore necessary to find some roentgenologic characteristics suggestive of malignancy. We found the following features useful as a practical guide:

1. Appearance of the base of the tumor.
2. Appearance of the surface of the tumor.
3. The size of the tumor.
4. The growth rate of the tumor.
5. The configuration of the tumor.

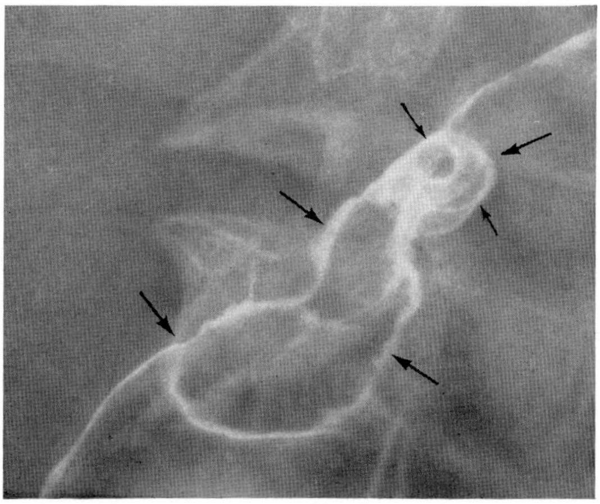

Fig. 34 b) ♂ 66 years. X-ray 14/8/62. A 30 mm long and 14 mm high polyp with typical indentation – cancer. Just proximal to that is a pedunculated polyp, 8 × 10 mm with the target phenomenon.

1. A morphologic change to which much importance must be attached is a constant dimpling or indentation at the base of the tumor, a small change that can be demonstrated only by the double contrast examination.
If a tangential view of a broad-based tumor shows such a constant indentation of the colonic wall at the site of the new formation, it is almost always a sign of invasive growth. By double contrast examination of rats with experimentally produced malignant tumors in the colon Rosengren (1973) found such an indentation in 100 percent. This change is perhaps not pathognomonic, because a local inflammatory process can, theoretically, also produce such a picture. This change is, however, so common in cancer that we regard it as an absolute indication for operation. But it should be observed that though such an indentation is important as a positive sign, its absence does not exclude the possibility of malignant degeneration. Such an indentation may also be seen in association with pedunculated polyps, but then it may be due simply to traction.
The indentation can be demonstrated in even very small tumors (Fig. 34a) and much more clearly in large ones (Fig. 34b). In such a picture there is no question that it is a real cancer.
2. Another morphologic feature, demonstrable only by the double contrast method, and useful in deciding whether a growth is malignant, is an irregular surface of the tumor (Fig. 35). Such a rough cauliflower-like surface instead of the smooth surface is statistically more frequent if the growth is malignant. But a smooth surface does not exclude the possibility of cancer.

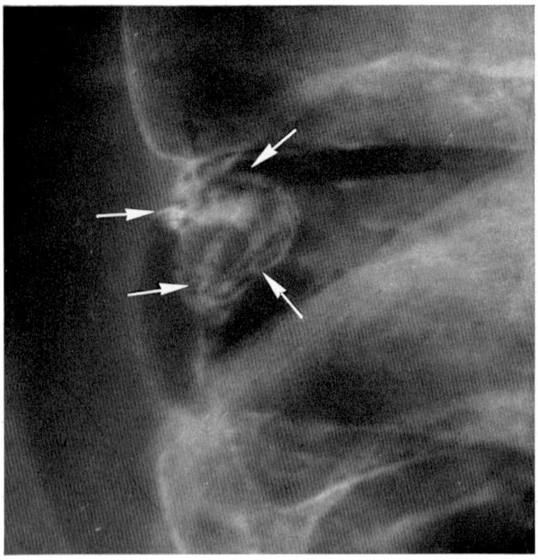

Fig. 35 ♂ 63 years. X-ray 25/4/53. Sessile polyp, 13 × 18 mm with irregular surface – malignant.

3. Analysis of the Malmö material has also shown that the size of a polypoid lesion is a significant physical characteristic. To form an opinion of the percentage of malignant and benign tumors and of the frequency of polyps with cellular atypia, in different sizes, 1,134 tumors were measured in roentgen films and after excision examined histologically. The results of this investigation are given in Table 6.

Table 6. Results of Histological Examination of Tumors

Size mm.	Cancer	Suspected Cancer	Atypical	Benign	Total
0– 5	3	6	250	165	424
	0.7%	1.4%	59%	38.9%	37.4%
6–10	8	36	124	153	321
	2.5%	11.2%	38.%	47.7%	28.3%
11–15	16	28	82	31	157
	10.2%	17.8%	52.5%	19.8%	13.8%
16–20	31	17	36	10	94
	33%	18.1%	38.3%	10.6%	8.3%
21–25	25	13	9	1	48
	52.1%	27.1%	18.8%	2.0%	4.2%
26–30	21	6	14	2	43
	48.8%	14.0%	32.6%	4.6%	3.8%
31–35	12	2	3	–	17
	70.6%	11.8%	17.6%		1.5%
35 <	25	2	3	–	30
	83.3%	6.7%	10.0%		2.7%
	141	110	521	362	1,134

It is clear from the table that even among the very small polypoid lesions (less than 5 mm in diameter) one must expect to find carcinomas with the same low age-specific incidence rates as those in the general population. The percentage of malignant polypoid lesions increases rapidly, while the benign neoplasms decrease in number. In this part of the material there were no benign lesions more than 30 mm in diameter.

This rule does not apply to children, in whom single or multiple polypoid lesions regularly exceed a diameter of 10 mm. The roentgenographic picture is one of benign tumors which may be followed up until they disappear or treatment is called for.

Measurements of fresh tissue specimens of a consecutive series of excised benign and malignant tumors showed that benign tumors rarely exceed 12 mm in diameter. Analysis of the diameters of 375 tumors in the Malmö material, measured in the first and the last film taken at serial double contrast examinations, showed the critical roentgenographic diameter to be 10 mm. The chances of a polypoid neoplasm more than 10 mm in diameter being malignant are so great, viz. 32 percent, that the size alone is sufficient to indicate surgical removal.

If the tumor is less than 10 mm in diameter and is of benign appearance, the patient should be kept under observation, re-examined every six months for the first two years and then at longer intervals. In view of the slow growth of such tumors, double contrast enema studies at shorter intervals are not necessary.

The importance of following up such patients is evident from the following set of roentgenograms (Fig. 36). – In November 1953 a 65-year-old man was referred for x-ray examination because of diffuse abdominal pain. Fig. 36a shows two polypoid lesions in the descending colon. The upper one is 5 by 8 mm and the lower 3 by 7 mm.

Six months later the polypoid tumor, situated higher up, had increased a little in size and was 9 by 7 mm in diameter (Fig. 36b).

In December 1954 both neoplasms were of the same size, but the upper one was now indented (Fig. 36c).

One year later check radiographs showed distinct progression both in the size of the tumor and of the indentation. The x-ray diagnosis was malignant tumor (Fig. 36d). The patient was operated upon, but the surgeon did not find the

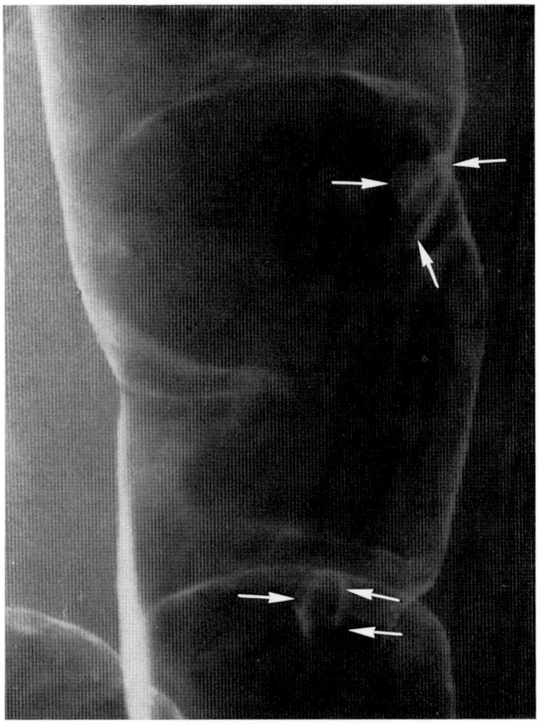

Fig. 36 ♂ 63 years. A follow-up patient.
a) X-ray 18/11/53. Two polyps in descending colon. The upper one is 5×8 mm.

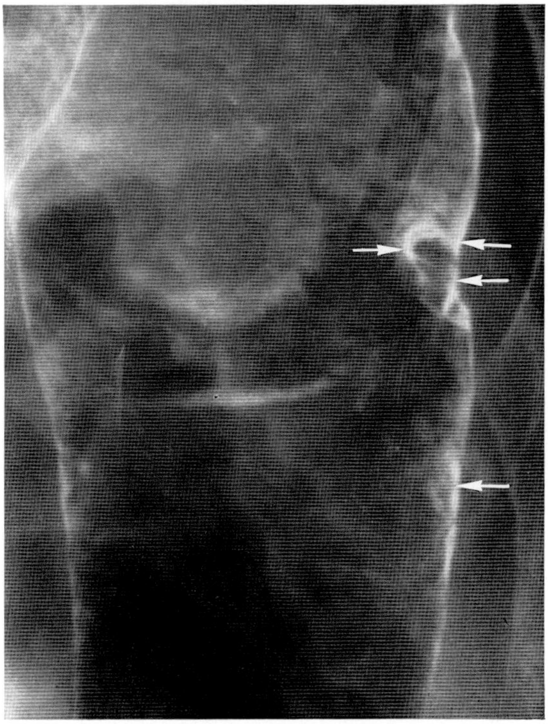

Fig. 36 b) X-ray 29/4/54. The upper one is now 7×9 mm.

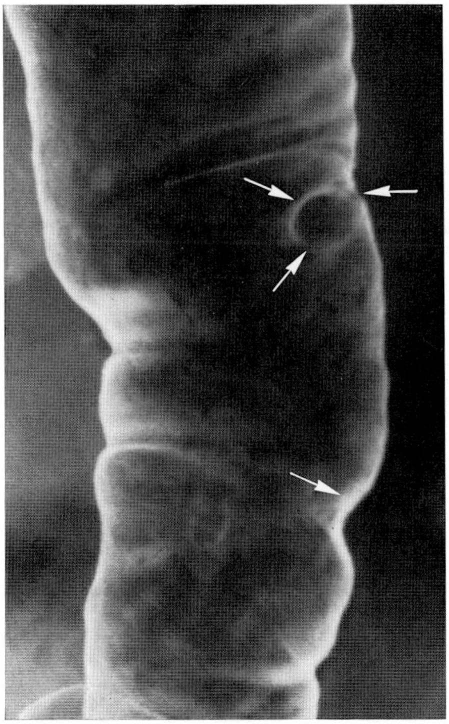

Fig. 36 c) X-ray 13/12/54. Same size.

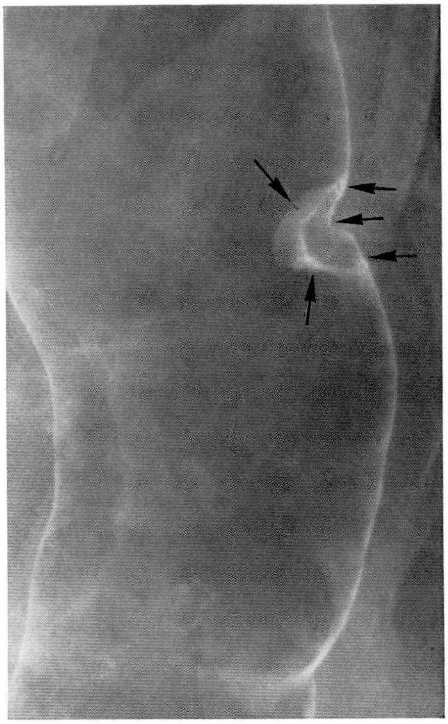

Fig. 36 d) X-ray 7/1/56. Increase in size of the upper one, now 10×11 mm. Typical indentation. Roentgen diagnosis: Cancer. Operation, but no palpable tumor and none seen despite colotomy and coloscopy.

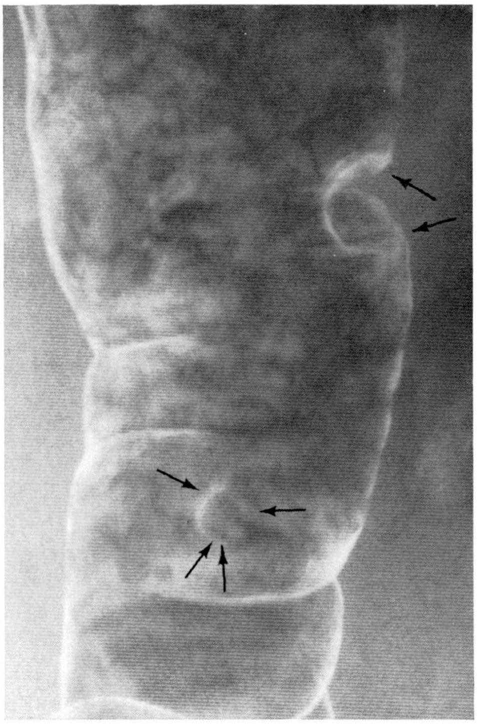

Fig. 36 e) X-ray 7/3/56. Control x-ray, Polyp still demonstrable.

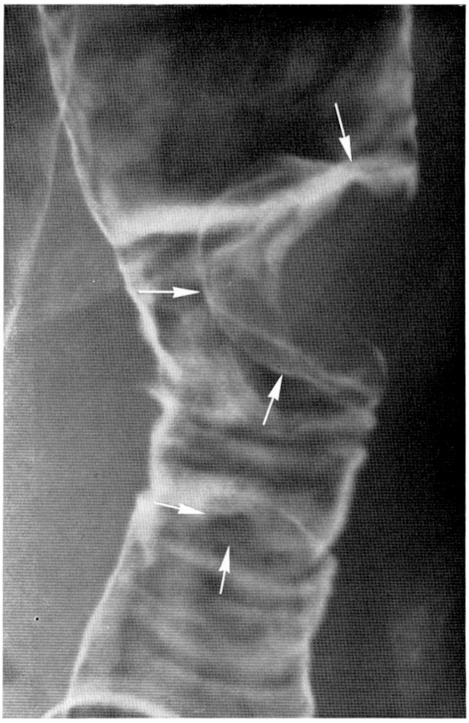

Fig. 36 f) X-ray 26/11/57. Large cancer. Livermetastases.

tumor despite palpation, colotomy and coloscopy.

At the re-examination two months later the polypoid lesion was still present and had grown a little in size, but the patient refused a new operation (Fig. 36e).

One-and-a-half years later, in May 1957, there was a large carcinoma (Fig. 36f). The patient was operated upon immediately, but the growth had spread to the liver.

4. Finally, the rate of the growth of these small tumors is very useful in the evaluation of malignancy. The rate of growth has always been a biologically important feature of all neoplasms. Though it has received extensive attention, nothing definite has so far been known about this rate in human beings.

In 1935 an English physiologist, Mottram, published an article "On the origin of tar tumors in mice, whether from single cell or many cells". He had found that the latent period between the application of tar and the appearance of epitheliomatous warts could be explained, if it was assumed that the tumors originated from single cells. He had also found that the tumors had very constant growth rates and that change in growth rate was rare.

An American scientist, Blum (1959), carried out similar experiments on rats. He used ultraviolet rays and measured the interval between the beginning of such irradiation and the appearance of cancer on the skin. He then measured the increase in size in relation to time and found that the tumors grow by geometric progression.

Collins (1956), followed the increase in the size of pulmonary metastases in human beings. He studied roentgenograms of the chest, taken at various intervals, of 22 patients with 24 pulmonary metastases from carcinoma of the colon and rectum. He found that pulmonary metastases grow by geometric progression and that the time necessary for a doubling of their volumes is a constant. Collins called this the "doubling time". It varied from case to case in his material but was much slower than he thought. The average doubling time was 116 days.

Collins then thought that the doubling time in a given case should be the same for the primary as for the secondary tumor, but that is not so. Most cancers of the colon and rectum grow over the mucosal surface of the bowel as circumferentially spreading plaques. It has therefore been possible to calculate the rate of growth from measurements made at repeated follow-ups. The plaques approach the geometric shape of cylinders until they achieve a diameter of several centimeters. At this stage some of them are prone to involve the entire circumference of the bowel – "napkin ring cancers". These surface-spreading growths remain fairly constant in thickness, and the changing volumes of the growing cancer are proportional to the surface areas, the latter being proportional to the squares of the diameters. Consequently, it is possible to regard the diameters, measured as the diameters of the bases of cylinders of uniform thickness, and in the calculation of experimental growth constants it is possible to regard surface areas as being proportional to volume. In accordance with this line Spratt and Ackerman in 1961 published one single case of carcinoma of the colon, which was observed by 9 double contrast enema studies over a seven-and-a-half year period. In this case the doubling time was 636 days. The outlines of 375 tumors in the Malmö double contrast roentgenograms, taken at repeated follow-ups, have also been measured. The patients had been examined on up to 10 occasions. The interval between the examinations was recorded in days. With the aid of data collected in this way, it was possible to define the changes in diameter over measured periods of time and to calculate the rate of growth. It may be pointed out that these measurements were made in roentgenograms. Thus the net results of the new cell formation, cell death, cell dissemination away from the primary tumors, and surface desquamation were measured. This cannot be done with any other method.

Statistical analysis of the findings made in the histologic sections of the tumors were classified by four pathologists and showed that the carcinomas were distinctly predominant in the more rapid range. The presence or absence of atypical changes in benign adenomatous polyps resulted in no change in the distribution of growth rates. This morphological alteration is probably of no consequence as far as rate of tumor is concerned. The "doubling time" of the invasively growing adenocarcinomas varied between 1,155 and 138 days. This corresponds to a linear-diametrical rate of growth between 0.003 and 0.025 mm/day. This rate is extremely slow.

From this calculation of the rate of growth it is also possible to calculate the risk of malignancy, and a statistical analysis showed that with a doubling time of more than 1,155 days the possibility of cancer is 1–2 percent. With a doubl-

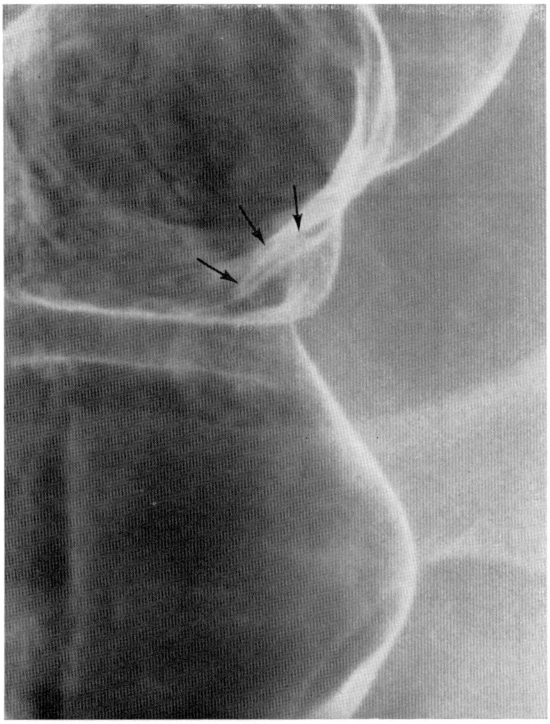

Fig. 37 a) ♂ 65 years. X-ray 39/1/56. Flat polyp, 2×13 mm. Cancer.

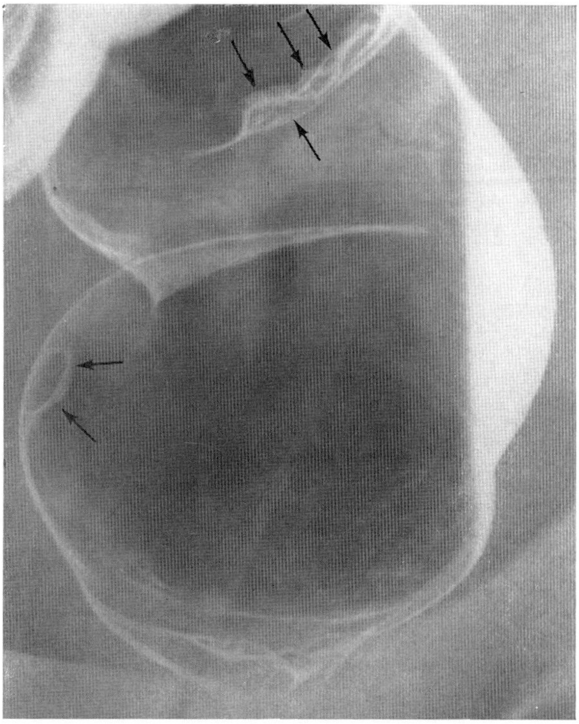

Fig. 37 b) ♂ 56 years. X-ray 21/11/63. 3×22 mm long sessile polyp along the fold of *Kohlrausch* – cancer.

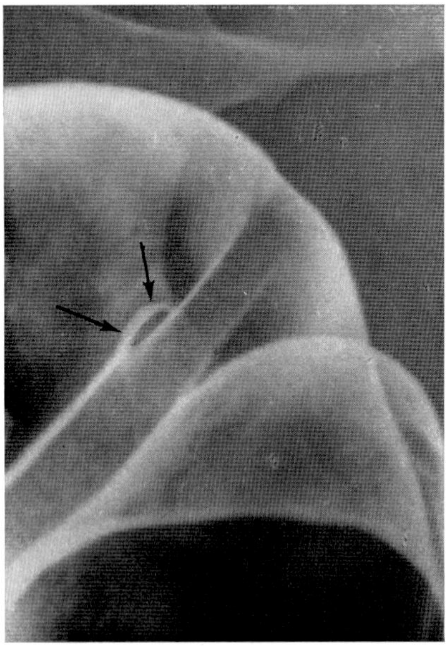

Fig. 33 ♀ 80 years:
a) X-ray 4/11/58. 3×7 mm sessile polyp along fold of Kohlrausch.

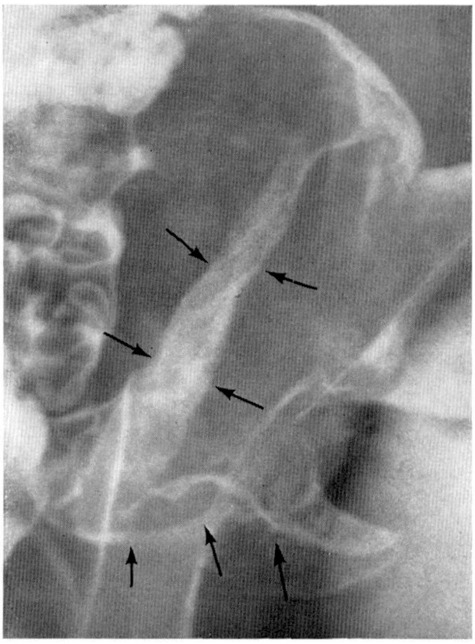

Fig. 38 b) Same patient. X-ray 7/7/64. Large cancer, infiltrating fold of Kohlrausch and right wall of the rectum.

ing time of 300–1,155 days it is 19–29 percent, but with a doubling time of less than 300 days the probability of the tumors being carcinomatous is 35 percent. One must therefore consider any increase in the size of a polypoid lesion as an absolute indication for operation.

5. In the evaluation of malignancy one can notice that when the breadth of the base of a polyp is greater than the height of the tumor in profile views, and the outline of the neoplasm in enface projection is oval – usually in transverse direction – the growth is more likely to be malignant (Figs. 37 a, b and 38 a, b).

Roentgenologic Indications for Operation

An analysis of the material has revealed certain definite indications for surgical intervention on polypoid tumors situated above the sigmoidoscopic level. The incidence of malignancy is much higher in these selected cases – 21 percent – than in those lesions of the rectum in which no selection is made (8 percent). The value of the roentgen signs is thus verified.

It is generally agreed that all polypoid lesions accessible by sigmoidoscopic vision should be removed transendoscopically, whether they produce symptoms or not and no matter how small they may be. The possibility of their being malignant is far too great to allow them to be left untreated. Their macroscopic appearance does not betray whether they are malignant. In addition, all workers in this field who regard polypoid lesions as premalignant or potentially malignant recommend their removal as a useful prophylactic measure.

In this connection it may be stressed that the rectum and the distal part of the sigmoid were formerly considered by the roentgenologists using the plain barium enema examination to be the most difficult parts of the colon to examine. Therefore they left this part to the sigmoidoscopists.

But with this new modification of the double contrast method this part of the colon is now the most adequately examined and therefore the double contrast method has become an excellent supplementary procedure to sigmoidoscopy, especially when the polypoid lesions are situated on the anterior wall above Houston's valves. The roentgen examination might thus precede sigmoidoscopy.

The roentgenographic indications for surgical removal of polyps above sigmoidoscopic levels are:

1. Signs of invasive growth at their base.
2. An irregular surface.
3. A diameter more than 10 mm.

4. An increase in size during follow-up.
5. Plateau-like configuration.
6. "Sentinel polyps".

We also recommend operation if roentgen examinations show multiple tumors. For it has been postulated that cancer is 5 times more common in patients with multiple polyps than in those with solitary polyps and that the frequency of cancer of the colon in patients with multiple polyps is about 20 percent.
In this connection the various syndromes associated with multiple polyps of the colon must be considered. Best known, because of the almost universal development of malignancy, is familial polyposis of the colon (Fig. 39). The diagnosis may be made by roentgen examination, which is especially important if sigmoidoscopy appears normal. The colon has a normal caliber and the walls are not rigid in the absence of malignant degeneration. This disease is transmitted by both sexes. About 50 percent of all offspring are affected, indicating a Mendelian dominance. Most of these patients contract an infiltrating carcinoma. For this reason prophylactic colectomy with an ileorectal anastomosis is usually recommended.
Isolated nonfamilial cases occur also with clinical and pathological features identical to those of the familial form.
"Sentinel polyps" are found in 15 percent of the operated cases of carcinoma of the colon in Malmö. In most of these cases the surgeons have not been able to palpate anything abnormal during the operation in that part of the colon where the sentinel polyps were situated. An x-ray examination with this modification is therefore necessary. Many of these polyps showed the same malignant histologic feature as the primary tumor. Of 124 patients in this material, who had been roentgenologically examined and operated upon and in whom sentinel polyps had been demonstrated and removed, the histological examination of these polyps in 19 (16 percent) of these cases showed cancer and in 129 marked atypical cells. Only 56 were stated to be nonmalignant, and in these cases the polyps were usually very small.
Sentinel polyps may be single or multiple and may occur far away from the primary tumor and still be malignant.
These findings stress how important it is to perform a double contrast examination even in cases with a large tumor so that the sentinel polyps may also be diagnosed. The surgeons feel it advisable to remove these polyps at the same time as the large tumor (Fig. 40).

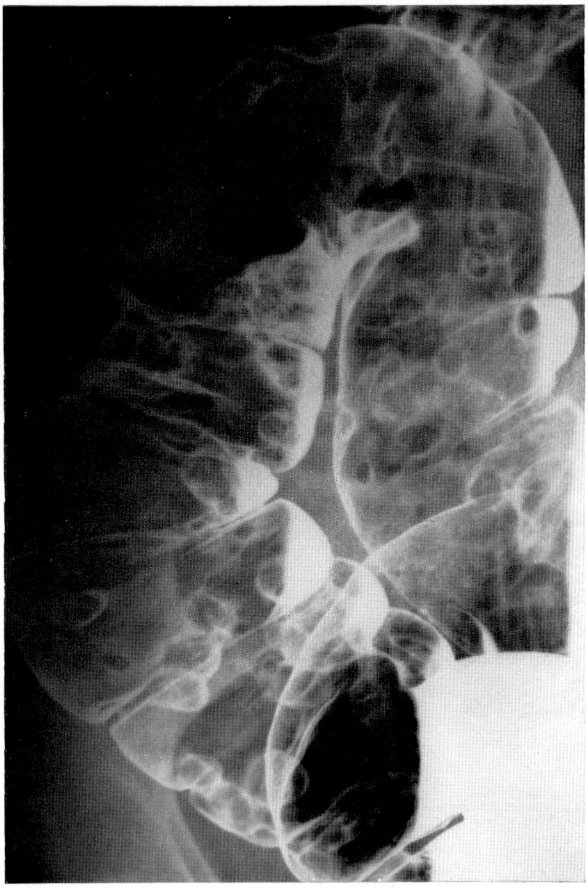

Fig. 39 ♀ 25 years. X-ray 21/8/59. Familial polyposis with multiple adenomata.

If the primary tumor completely obstructs the intestine, the patient is examined as soon as possible after the operation for the purpose of finding any sentinel polyps.
It must also be stressed that if the sentinel polyps are not removed immediately, it is necessary to follow up these polyps also. Fig. 41 demonstrates this.
A roentgen examination in August 1955 showed diverticula in the sigmoid and a complete obstruction with a cancer-typical border with shelving and irregularity in the descending colon (Fig. 41a). At the operation the surgeons were not able to palpate anything abnormal in the proximal part of the colon.
A control examination one year later showed a polypoid lesion in the ascending colon but no operation was performed (Fig. 41b).

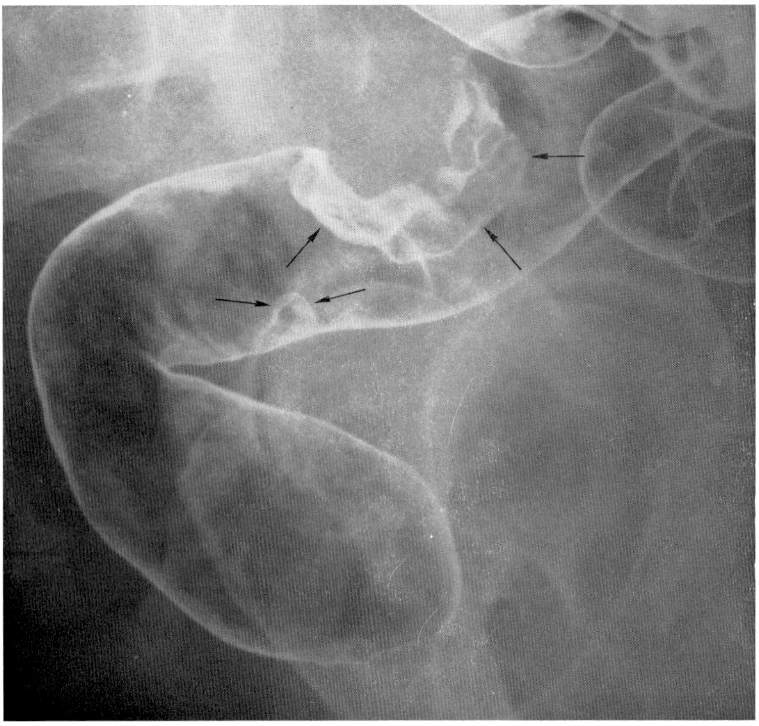

Fig. 40 ♂ 74 years. X-ray 2/4/58. Large rectal cancer on posterior wall with sentinel polyp.

At a further follow-up examination 2 years later the polyp was wrongly reported to be of the same size (Fig. 41 c). Four years later a large tumor was present at the same site. The patient was immediately operated upon and a carcinoma was removed (Fig. 41 d).

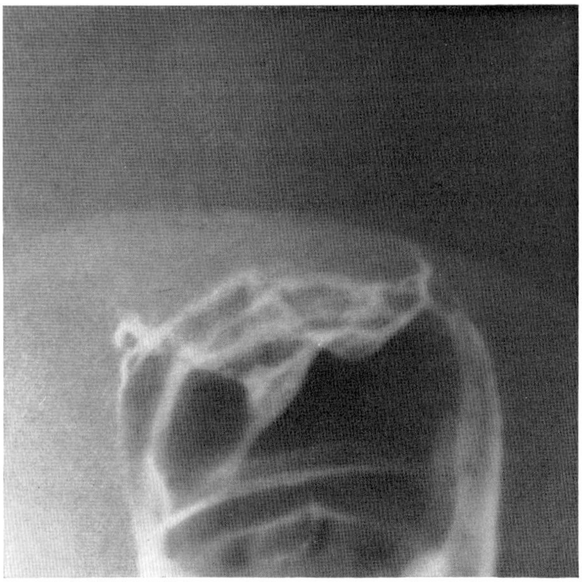

Fig. 41 ♀ 69 years. A follow-up patient:
a) X-ray 4/8/55. Completely obstructing cancer of descending colon.

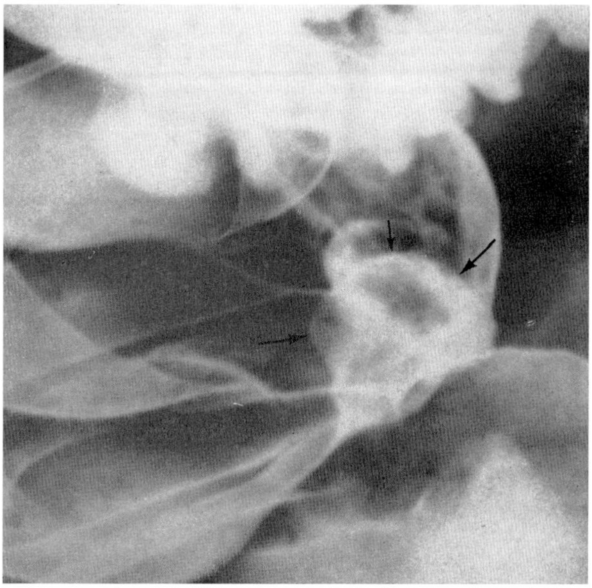

Fig. 41 b) X-ray 22/8/56. Sentinel polyp in the ascending colon, 15×15 mm. The patient refused surgery.

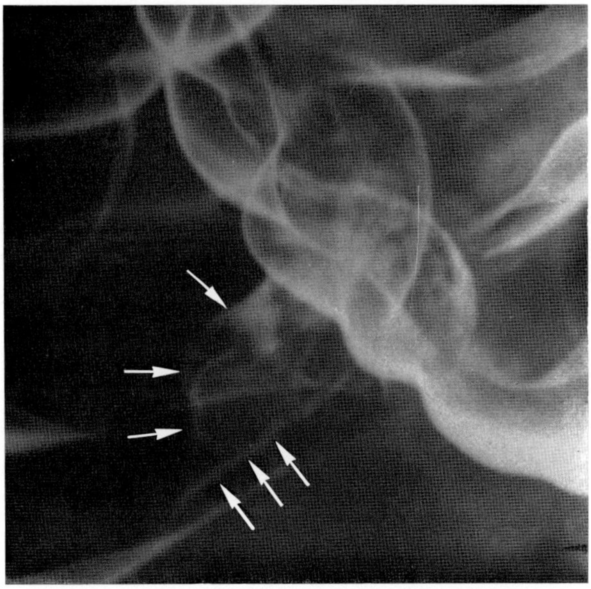

Fig. 41 c) X-ray 14/5/58. The polyp increased to 15×38 mm but urgery was still refused.

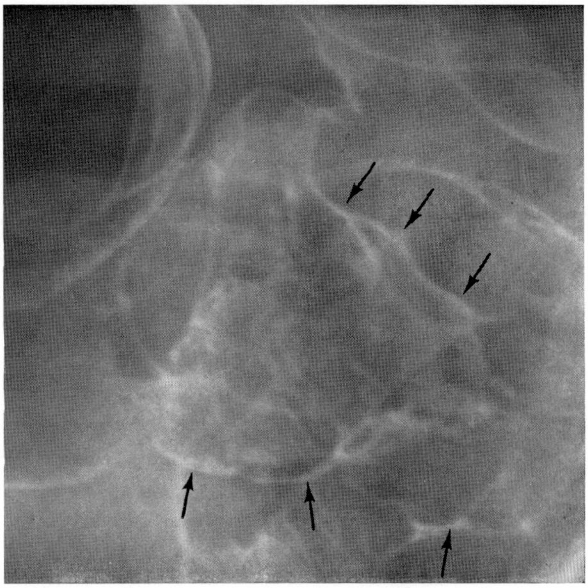

Fig. 41 d) X-ray 11/1/62. Now a large carcinoma.

Follow-up

To facilitate a follow-up of these patients a special unit has been set up at the hospital. The patients are referred for first check roentgenography within 3 months of the operation and later annually, or, if necessary, also at shorter intervals. The purpose of the follow-up is to observe the polypoid neoplasms which were less than 10 mm at the first roentgen examination and showed no signs of malignancy and were therefore not excised. The second purpose is to visualize the margins of the segment excised. In the latter cases the first examination after operation is very important if the cut surfaces lie above the reach of the sigmoidoscope. This examination gives a postoperative base-line and the examination can then tell us in the future which changes are due to surgery and which are due to recurrent neoplasm. Recurrences which may be due to malignant cells left behind at the surgical operation, development of predisposing cells, degeneration of sentinel polyps or of implantation of tumor cells at the actual operation, usually occur as irregularities in the outline of the mucosa (Fig. 42a, b) and later as unilateral or circular stenosis. From a differential diagnostic point of view in the early cases one must also bear in mind the possibility of granuloma due to a foreign body reaction.

Results

The vital question is whether removal of the small malignant and pre-malignant polypoid neoplasms is early enough, i.e. before metastases have developed. At a follow-up of 1,106 patients operated on for polyps in Malmö, including 141 with fully developed cancer histologically and 637 with more or less marked atypical cells, only 2 patients have developed metastases, as far as we know. The oldest cases were followed for up to 10 years. In one patient the polyp was 22 by 22 mm. This patient never complied with our request for a repeat examination. Four years after roentgen examination the patient was admitted to our hospital in a severely cachectic condition and died from gastrointestinal bleeding before roentgenography could be performed. Autopsy revealed a large cancer at the site of the previously diagnosed polyp and liver metastases. In the other case, where the excised polyp was 25 by 30 mm, the patient died suddenly 1 year after the operation. He also had liver metastases.

Besides these two patients there were two others, one in whom the surgeon at operation was unable to find the malignant polyp illustrated in the roentgenogram (Fig. 36), and the other a patient who had either misunderstood his doctor or did not wish to be operated on. He came back four years after the roentgen examination and had

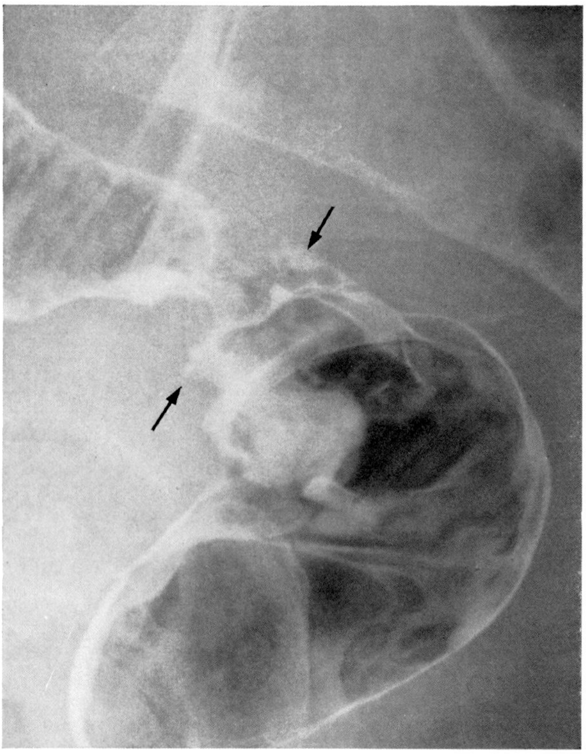

Fig. 42 ♀ 50 years. Cancer resection:
a) X-ray 6/12/56. Anastomosis with smooth contours.

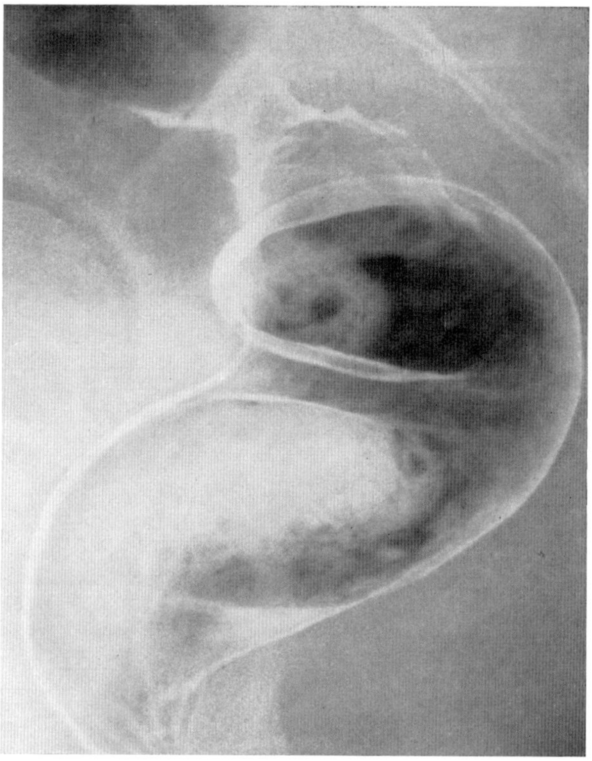

Fig. 42 b) X-ray 21/1/57. Now irregular contours recurrence.

a large annular cancer 4 cm long at the site of the polyp.

Some other investigators in this field also found that metastases are very rare. It has therefore been claimed that these polypoid tumors, which histologically look like cancer, do not behave like biologically true cancer, and that the roentgen diagnosis of these small polypoid lesions is of no significance. Experience gained with this material, however, argues strongly against such a view. There are thus cases of large carcinoma of the colon, in which earlier double contrast films are available for comparison. In 45 cases with annular cancer, a polypoid lesion at the same site was detected by reviewing earlier double contrast films. In all these cases the diagnosis at the previous examination was *no* tumor. But on later examination of the earlier films, which had, as a rule, been taken some years previously, polypoid formations were seen with signs of malignancy at the same site as the present cancer. These cases show that an early diagnosis and early surgical intervention are of great importance.

There has been a steady rise in the frequency of death from cancer of the large bowel in all countries, and in the United States, for example, cancer of colon and rectum has been claiming more deaths than cancer of any other organ. The mortality has increased steadily with advancing age, especially in urban populations. According to the American Cancer Society in 1965 as many as 73,000 persons were found to have cancer of the rectum and colon. Of these 43,000 died from the disease.

In Great Britain the number of deaths from cancer of the colon and rectum in 1963 was 14,426 and the large intestine is probably the site of more cancers than any other organ.

In Sweden in 1962 cancer of the colon and rectum was diagnosed in 2,622 patients, which means 11.8 percent of all cases of cancer found in that country.

The disease is thus very common, and it is apparent from the American figures that the results of treatment are far from satisfactory. Though cancer of the colon does not belong to the most malignant types of cancer, though it

sets up secondaries relatively late, and though it has a fairly good prognosis if operated upon in time, the 5-year survival rate is still very discouraging because so many cases are inoperable by the time they are diagnosed.
Since the etiology of the disease is still obscure despite intense research, no real prophylactic measures are available; the only thing we can do to improve the results is to try to get as early a diagnosis as possible and an early operation. This modification of the double contrast method is hence of great importance.

Polyps in Children

Polyps in children deserve special mention. Yates (1953) states that they differ in two respects from those in adults: in children they are rarely malignant and, secondly, they often disappear spontaneously. The polyps are usually pedunculated and may be solitary, clustered or disseminated. They are more frequently solitary than multiple. The ratio of pedunculated to broad-based polyps is said to be 3:1.
According to Helwig (1946) the frequency of polyps found at autopsy of children is 3 percent, while Horilleno (1957) gives only 0.075 percent. The frequency in a series examined with the double contrast method is naturally much higher, since it is a selected material. In the Malmö patients below 20 years of age the frequency of polyps is 19.2 percent during the first decade and 8.2 percent during the second. According to Kerr (1948) one-third of all polyps are situated above sigmoidoscopic level. Wolf and co-workers (1961) give a frequency of 10 percent for this group.

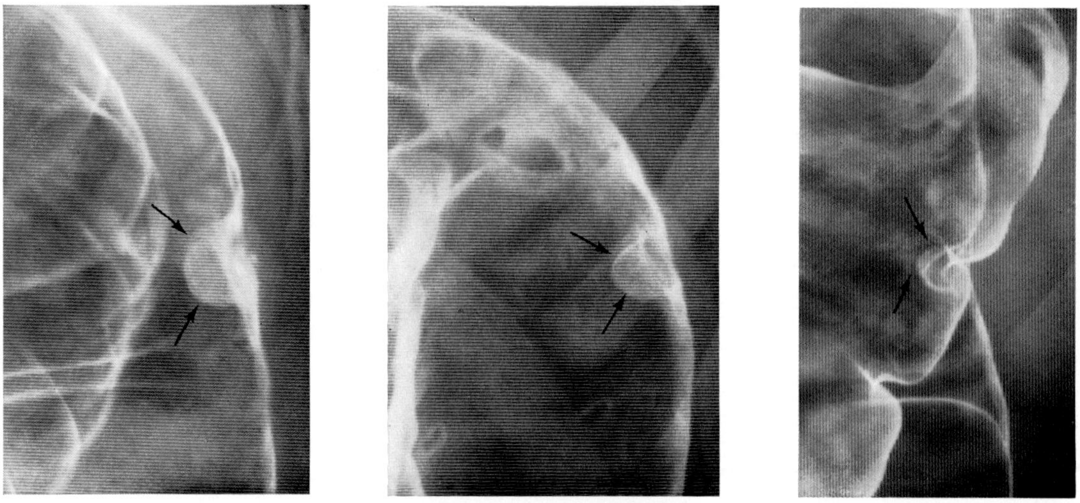

a b c

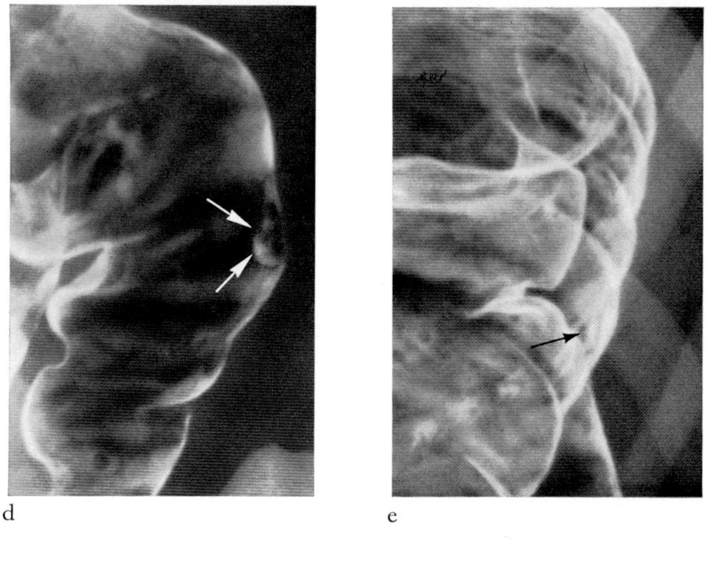

d e

Fig. 43 ♀ 5 years. A follow-up patient:
a) X-ray 21/11/53. Sessile polyp in descending colon, 10×10 mm.
b) X-ray 11/8/55. The polyp has decreased to 7×7 mm.
c) X-ray 7/1/56. Polyp still decreasing, now 3×6 mm.
d) X-ray 16/8/57. 3×4 mm.
e) X-ray 10/2/58. 1×3 mm.

Many pathologists share the view that polyps are of the same type in children as in adults, but, according to Harris (1953), the histologic picture of polyps in children suggests a much higher degree of activity. Some authors have also described a frequently multiple juvenile type, whose appearance is characterized not only by its adenomatous structure, but also by cyst-like glands and cellular infiltration with eosinophilic cells. These juvenile polyps are seldom malignant. Schille (1954) reported one malignant case in a 2-year-old child. We have never seen such a case in Malmö.

According to Curry (1954), polyps can occur in 6-month-old children. At autopsy of 499 subjects below 21 years, however, Helwig could not demonstrate any polyps in children below 1 year. It is generally claimed that most polyps are diagnosed within the first decade of life – especially between the third and fifth year – seldom during the second decade, but afterwards with increasing frequency between the ages of 20 and 30 (Scarborough, 1965). According to Hughes and Jenkins (1956), this may be explained by spontaneous shedding of these neoplasms, especially in children. Judging from our experience, it would seem that the low frequency of polyps in the latter part of childhood can also be explained by spontaneous regression of the growths. At follow-up of our patients we have found that the sessile polyps sometimes disappear completely. An example of such regression is given below.

A 5-year-old girl was referred for roentgen examination of the colon because of intestinal bleeding. Examination in November 1953 revealed one 10 by 10 mm rectal polyp, which was extirpated, and one polyp in the distal limb of the splenic flexure. This polypoid formation also measured 10 by 10 mm on the x-ray film (Fig. 43a).

The girl was examined again in August 1955 because of abdominal pain. The polyp measured 7 by 7 mm. (Fig. 43b).

In January 1956 the patient again had abdominal pain, but no diarrhea or melena. Re-examination showed that the tumor had become smaller and was 3 by 6 mm (Fig. 43c).

Re-examination in August 1957 because of abdominal pain in the region of the umbilicus showed further regression of the tumor (Fig. 43d). In February 1958 it was still smaller and then measured only 1 by 3 mm (Fig. 43e).

The commonest cause of intestinal bleeding in children is polypoid neoplasms. Other symptoms produced by such neoplasms are watery and often blood-stained stools, as well as protrusion of the polyp through the anus. If the polyp is situated further up the intestine, it may cause abdominal pain, presumably because of temporary invagination; the clinical picture may then sometimes resemble ulcerative colitis.

Treatment is surgical, but the observation of spontaneous regression means that demonstration of a polyp does not indicate immediate operation; one can and ought to postpone operation unless it is indicated by rectal bleeding or other symptoms.

7 Villous Tumors

Introduction

The villous tumor is an established clinicopathologic entity and the name is appropriate for those tumors which do not conform to the classical appearance of the adenomatous growth pattern. According to Wood (1972), these tumors fall largely into the following three groups according to their gross appearance:

1. A flat carpet-like growth, which is frequently very extensive in both the longitudinal and circumferential measurements. It may resemble congenital polyposis of the more common adenomatous variety.

2. The second and most common type has a central irregularity and consists of a poorly demarcated bulky mass, composed of small fingerlike villi or fronds, separated from each other by deep clefts, giving an appearance resembling "bouquets". They generally assume a cauliflower-like fungating appearance. Carpet-like growth may extend for some distance beyond the more central and bulkier lesion.

3. The third type, constituting about 10 percent of all villous tumors, has a short broad pedicle which is the result of mechanical adjustments during contraction of the wall of the colon.

The villous tumors thus generally have a very characteristic gross appearance and arise from the mucous membrane, attached to the wall by a broad base. This is, however, not true if they occur in the pure polypoid form.

They vary in size from a few millimeters up to 15 to 20 cm and may involve the entire circumference of the intestinal wall. They are often more than 5 cm in diameter before they are detected. They are raised about 1 to 3 cm above the surrounding mucosa and often show focal areas of hemorrhage or ulceration on their surface. They are usually single, but may be multiple. They have a soft plush-like consistency and can easily escape palpation by the examining finger.

Villous tumors occur equally often in both sexes and are most common in the sixth and seventh decades. The patients are thus usually older than those with other types of epithelial growths of the large intestine.

The quotient between the incidence of these small tumors and all tumors of the large bowel has been given as 1.4 percent by Sunderland and Binkley (1948), 2.3 percent by Bacon (1951) and 1.85 percent by Hines et al. (1958). Figures up to 15 percent have also been published. Wood (1972) says that these tumors are about one-fifth as common as those of the adenomatous polypoid type. They may therefore be regarded as fairly rare.

The tumors occur principally in the rectum and sigmoid and are uncommon in the right and transverse colon. A summary of the literature shows that approximately 90 percent occur in the rectum and sigmoid and 10 percent in the descending, transverse and ascending colon.

The relationship to colonic cancer makes the lesions of major clinical significance.

Hines found that 8 percent of villous tumors of the rectum showed signs of invasive carcinoma. Sunderland and Binkley found malignant degeneration in 68.7 percent of their cases; 39.5 percent being invasive carcinoma. Some reports give an even higher frequency of malignant transformation – 74 percent (Swinton, 1939 and Wheat and Ackerman 1958). Malignant change in this originally benign tumor is thus not only common, but is to be expected. According to some authors malignant changes are more common in the larger lesions and the size of the lesions is the most significant feature in estimating whether or not malignancy is present. According to Kaye and Bragg (1968), 91 percent of villous tumors less than 5 cm in diameter are benign and two-thirds of the villous adenomas of 8 cm or more show invasive carcinoma. Turek (1971) found that 25 percent of lesions smaller than 2 cm in diameter have invasive carcinoma, but that size alone is not sufficient to decide whether a lesion is malignant.

In the early benign stages the tumor involves only the mucosa and is readily movable over the muscularis through the submucosa, but invasive carcinoma alters the nature of the tumor. There is then a typical hard, indurated, fairly well demarcated and possibly ulcerated lesion. In many instances it is apparent that malignant areas have penetrated the deeper levels, and they are a known forerunner of colonic carcinoma.

Histologically, the villous tumors have been subdivided into 4 groups (Wheat and Ackerman).

1. Villous adenomas that appear to be completely benign.
2. Villous adenomas with areas that show focal atypical changes. These are small focal areas, where there is stratification of the lining epithelial cells, some loss of nuclear polarity, and intraglandular budding. These cells also stain more intensely than the surrounding cells.
3. Villous adenomas with focal carcinoma. These tumors may have focal atypical changes, but they also show small focal areas of carcinoma strictly limited to the mucosa (formerly called carcinoma in situ).
4. These are villous adenomas with invasive carcinoma.

There are probably no very reliable clinical criteria for evaluating malignant degeneration or malignant change, but increasing rectal bleeding may certainly herald a malignant change in the tumor. Alterations found by palpation, such as increased resistance or fixation or ulceration are significant, and certainly suggest the possibility of malignancy.

In the individual case it is safest to assume that any given villous tumor is cancerous until extensive histologic study has shown that it is not.

Symptoms

Small villous tumors are usually asymptomatic, and they may attain considerable size before bleeding or other symptoms appear. The larger lesions, however, produce a wide range of symptoms. The most common clinical manifestation (in about one-third of the patients) is the passage of copious amounts of mucus through the anus. This is called pseudo- or mucous diarrhea, which may cause remarkable fluid and electrolytic disturbances. The diarrhea is rarely associated with tenesmus or pain, for this tumor is rarely painful. Bleeding is not unusual. It is more commonly seen after premalignant or definitely ulcerative and malignant changes have occurred.

The tumors sometimes produce a feeling of fullness or a feeling that the rectum is not properly empty after defecation, which results in some change in normal bowel habit. Fragments of the tumor and bits of tissue frequently are passed, which are referred to as "free biopsies". Even very large tumors rarely cause obstructive symptoms. This is because the bowel tends to dilate to accommodate the presence of the very bulky mass.

Villous tumors occurring higher up the colon – and they may occur in any portion of the colon – cause symptoms slightly different from those in the rectum proper, viz. the occurrence of mucus, usually in large quantities, and minor bleeding, because there is less direct trauma due to hard stools and because the rectal tumors have a tendency to prolapse.

Clinical Diagnosis

Early diagnosis of these potentially malignant tumors is important. According to many clinicians, half of all villous tumors that feel soft on palpation, and all of those that feel hard, are malignant. The importance of careful palpation, sigmoidoscopic examination and of a double contrast study cannot be overemphasized.

Roentgen Diagnosis

Despite the characteristic gross features only little attention has hitherto been paid to the possibility of roentgen diagnosis. This was because the results obtained with the conventional barium enema were far from satisfactory. Aurin and Marietta (1961) claimed that the barium enema was useless, and Hines was able to make a preoperative diagnosis in only 2 out of 71 cases. Frye (1952), however, who described one case of villous tumor of the sigmoid, stated that the roentgenogram with the sharply demar-

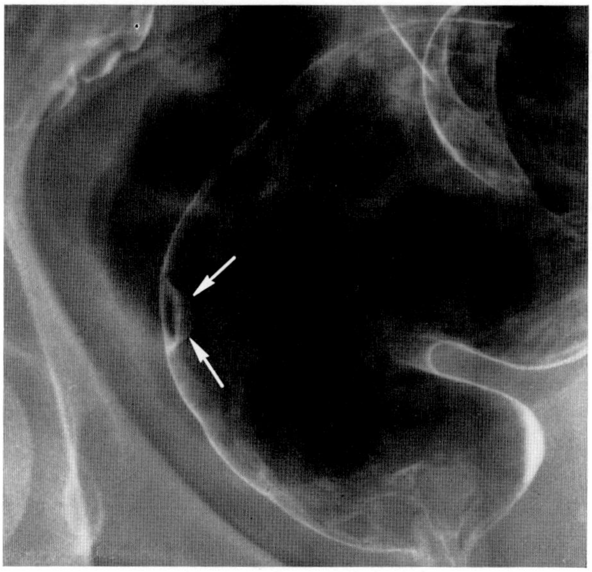

Fig. 44 ♀ 72 years:
a) X-ray 2/1/59. Intermediate polyp in rectum. 7×12mm.

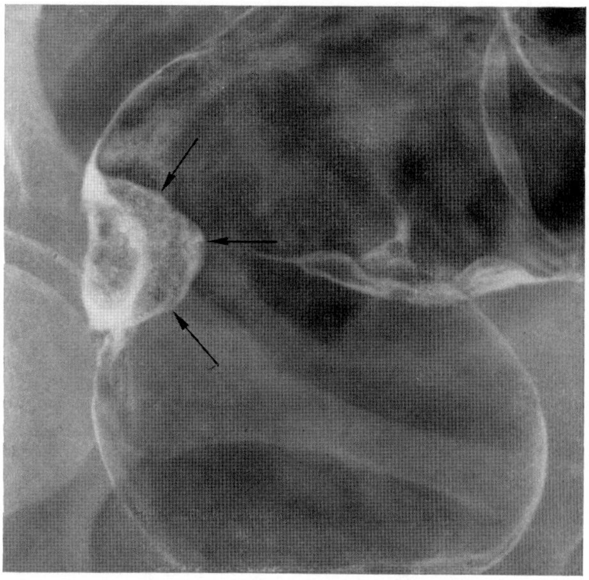

Fig. 44 c) Oblique view at same examination revealed typical indentation. Malignant.

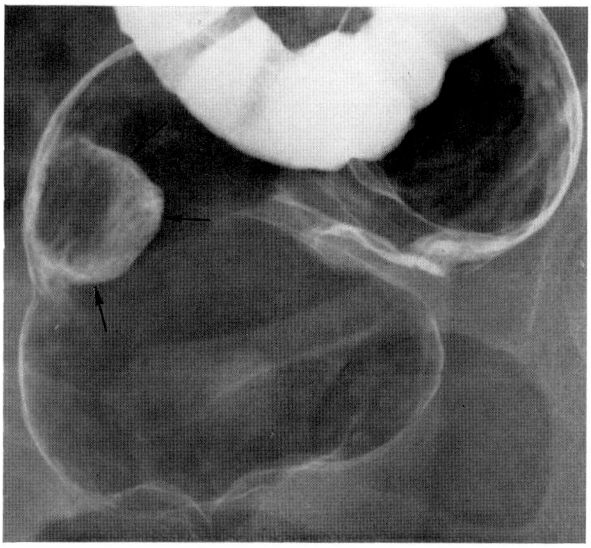

Fig. 44 b) Same patient. X-ray 10/3/61. Increased size of polyp, now 22×23 mm.

cated mass, into which extended linear streaks of barium apparently between the mucus-covered folds and villi of the tumor, was characteristic. He had also observed that following evacuation the tumor appeared to be reduced in size with a rough, serrated feathery margin. He attributed this reduction in size to the expulsion, on evacuation, of the large quantity of mucus produced and collected within the tumor. Wolf (1960) reported that the large villous tumors showed fairly distinct filling defects at the beginning of the infusion of the barium enema but that they afterwards disappeared. Wolf also claimed that the tumors could be diagnosed in the postevacuation films and in the double contrast roentgenograms.

The introduction of this modification of the double contrast method with its capability to depict the mucosa in detail and demonstrate even very small changes, considerably improved our diagnostic possibilities. In Malmö, for example, all surgically treated patients with villous tumors are diagnosed by preoperative roentgen examination after the introduction of our modification.

The appearance of the villous tumors in the double contrast roentgenograms varies widely. Sometimes they assume the form of small solitary broad-based polyps with an even and smooth outline and with a diameter of less than 1 cm (Fig. 44a). In such cases they cannot, of course, be differentiated from adenomatous polyps. They sometimes retain their polyp-like configuration even when they have assumed a diameter of more than 20 mm (Fig. 44b, c).

Sometimes the outline is irregular, papillary, cauliflower like, and even then they cannot be distinguished from an adenoma (Fig. 45a).

Sometimes the villous papilloma is pedunculated and of irregular outline but no differential diagnosis is possible as the pedunculated adeno-

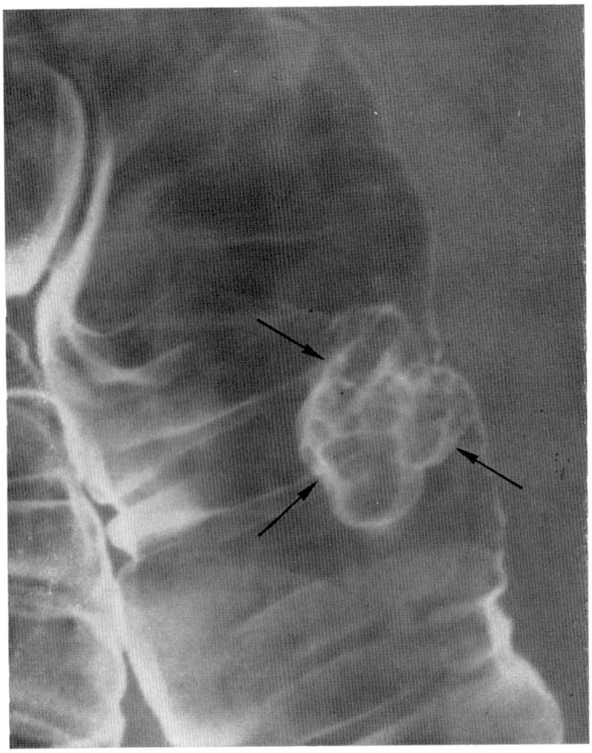

Fig. 45 a) ♀ 74 years. X-ray 5/1/61. Typical villous papilloma in transverse colon.

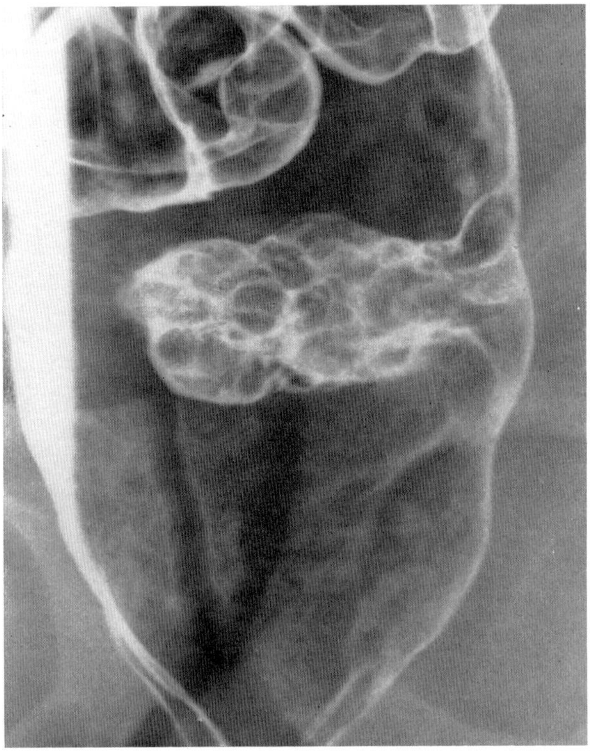

Fig. 45 b) ♂ 70 years. X-ray 12/9/57. Typical villous papilloma in the rectum.

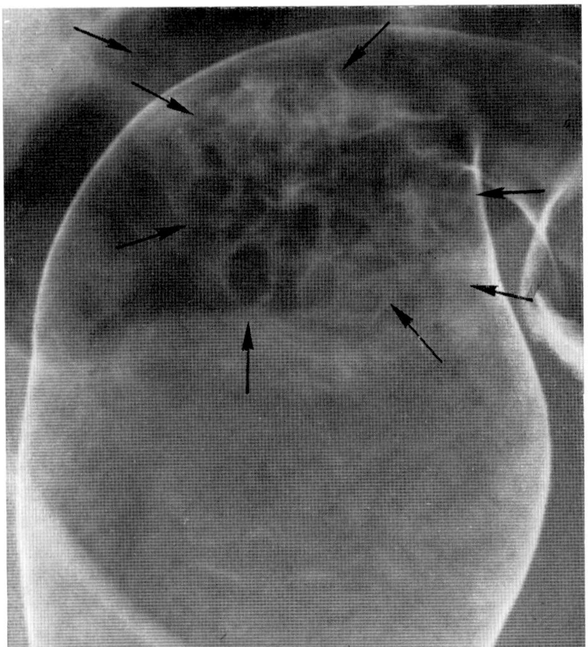

Fig. 46 ♀ 80 years. X-ray 6/8/62. Typical flat villous papilloma of rectum.

mas may have a similar surface. But the large pedunculated villous papillomas (Fig. 45b) often have a very characteristic and readily recognized appearance and in these cases there are usually no difficulties in making a differential diagnosis from a pedunculated adenomatous polyp.

In other cases the villous papilloma is flat. They are often several centimeters in diameter before the patients are referred for roentgen examination. The changes are confined to a distinct area where the normal mucosal relief is entirely destroyed. The roentgenograms show different-sized crowded defects. They give the change a "cobblestone" appearance and the spongy structure varies with the distance between the individual villi or villi in groups (Fig. 46).

Tangential views reveal changes usually barely a centimeter in depth and the surface is often irregular (Figs. 48 and 50b).

Another characteristic of the villous papilloma is that since it is soft it can change in size and shape with the degree of insufflation of the intes-

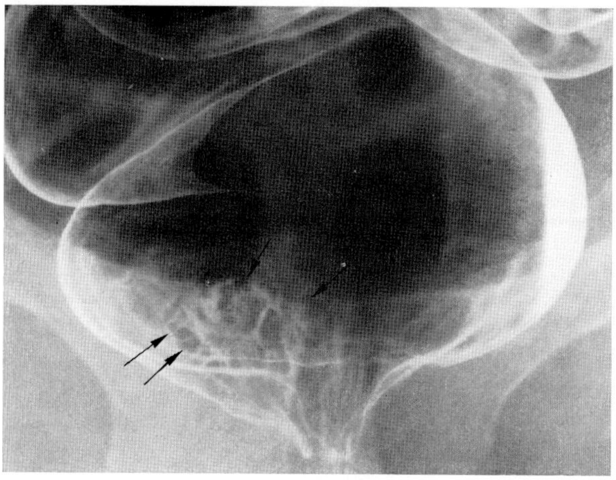

a

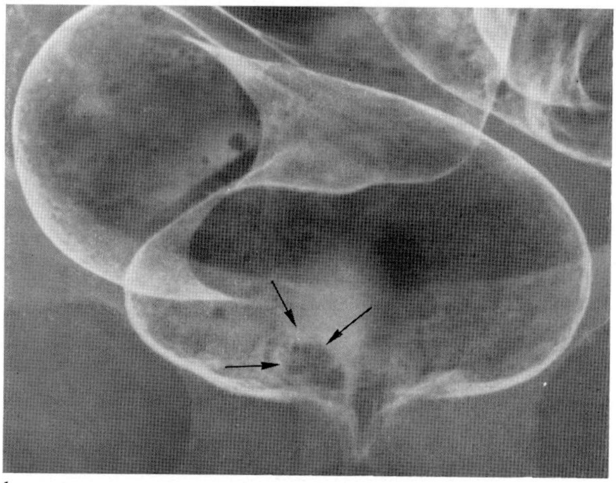

b

Fig. 47 ♀ 68 years. X-ray 6/8/56. a), b) Variation in size and configuration during the same examination.

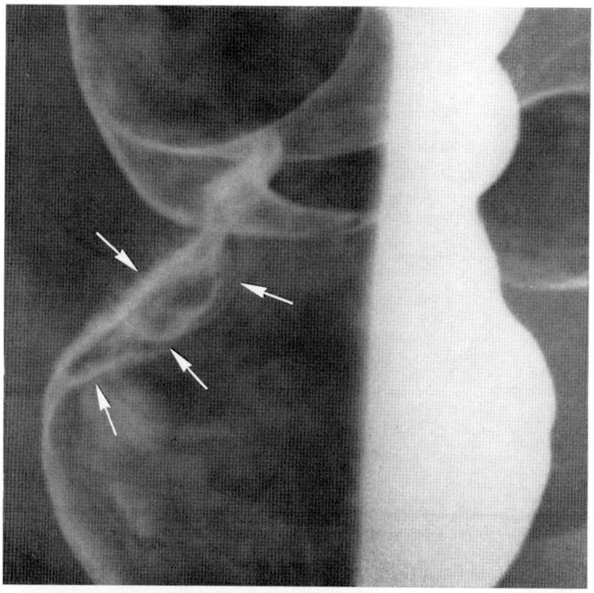

tine during one and the same examination (Figs. 47a, b).

Another fairly common characteristic is the shagginess of its outline (Fig. 48).

Recurrences are common and the patients, like those with adenoma, should therefore be regularly followed up (Figs. 49a, b).

As for the possibilities of diagnosing the malignancy roentgenologically, Wolf claimed that ulcerations and an irregular, unchanging outline suggest malignancy. Other authors do not believe that it is possible to judge the outline roentgenologically.

Judging from our experience in Malmö, the

Fig. 48 ♂ 70 years. X-ray 7/1/57. Typical contour of a villous papilloma in oblique view.

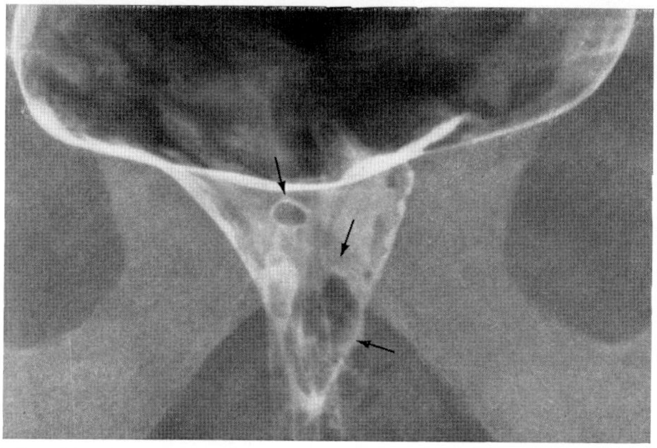

Fig. 49 ♀ 68 years. Operated upon in July 58 for villous papilloma in the rectum:
a) X-ray 17/10/58. Small recurrence. Operated upon again.

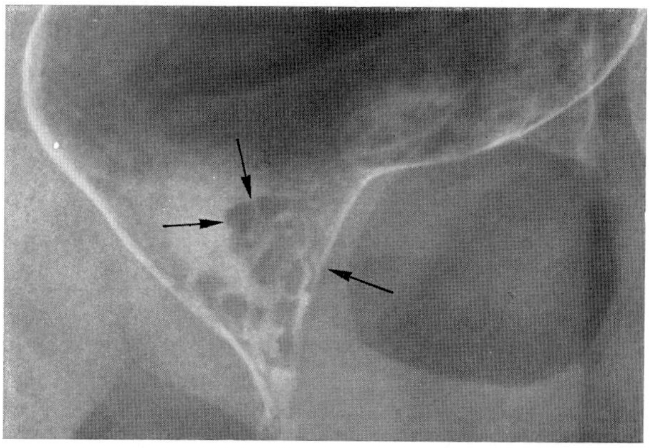

Fig. 49 b) X-ray 1/6/60. Control examination. New recurrence.

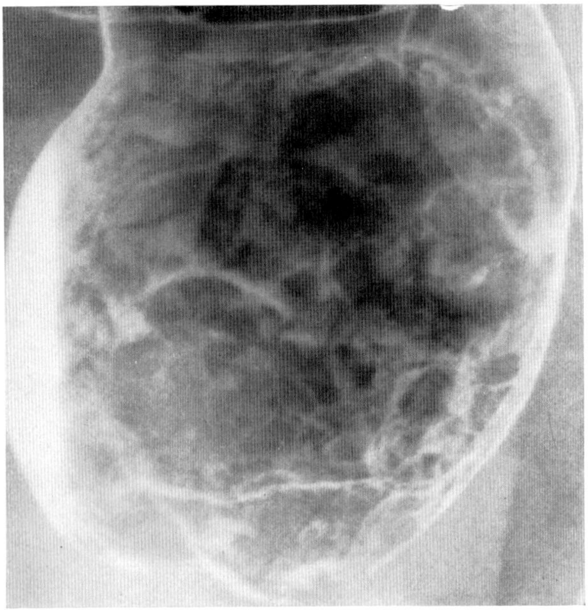

Fig. 50 ♂ 73 years. X-ray 17/11/56:
a) Frontal view. Very large typical villous adenoma of rectum. Clinical diagnosis: proctitis.

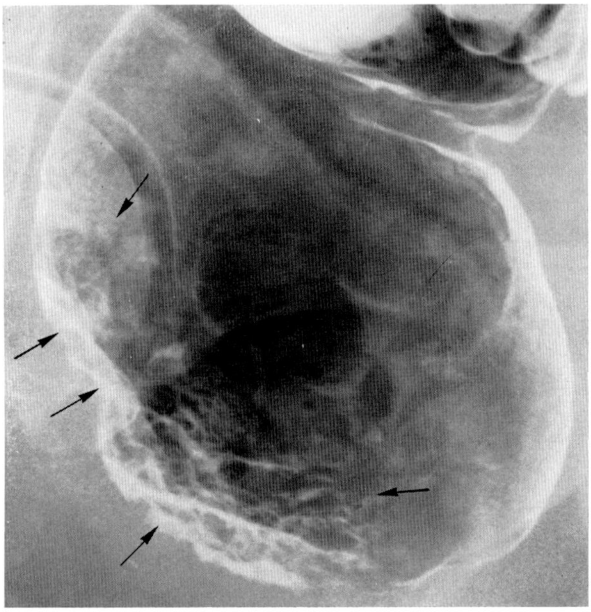

Fig. 50 b) Oblique view. Relatively flat tumor with indentation.

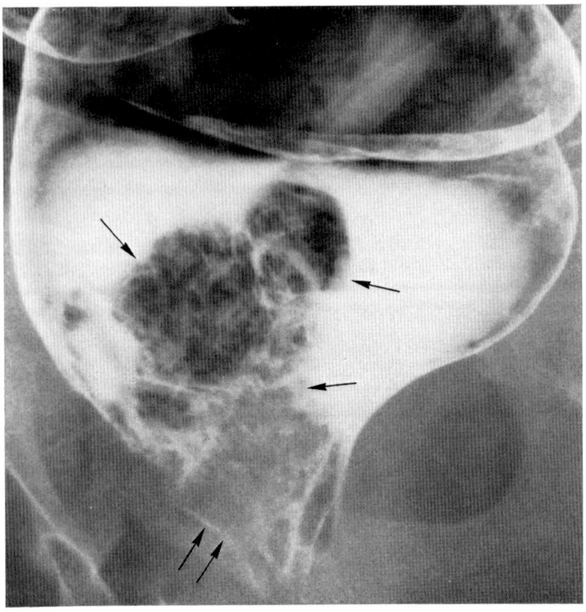

Fig. 51 ♀ 68 years. X-ray 15/7/58:
a) Frontal view. Large villous papilloma of rectum.

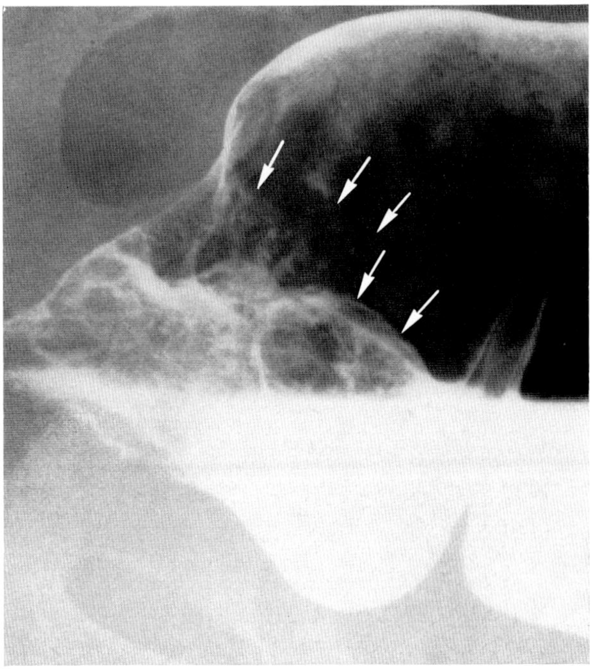

Fig. 51 b) In left recumbent position, the tumor is in the same position.

double contrast method in most cases permits a diagnosis of malignancy. For a malignant villous papilloma often exhibits indentation of its base. This characteristic change was found in all our malignant cases, but not in any of the benign ones. One might therefore wonder whether this characteristic roentgenographic sign alone might not be sufficient to indicate radical operation regardless of the results of the histologic examination of biopsy specimens. Such indentation is

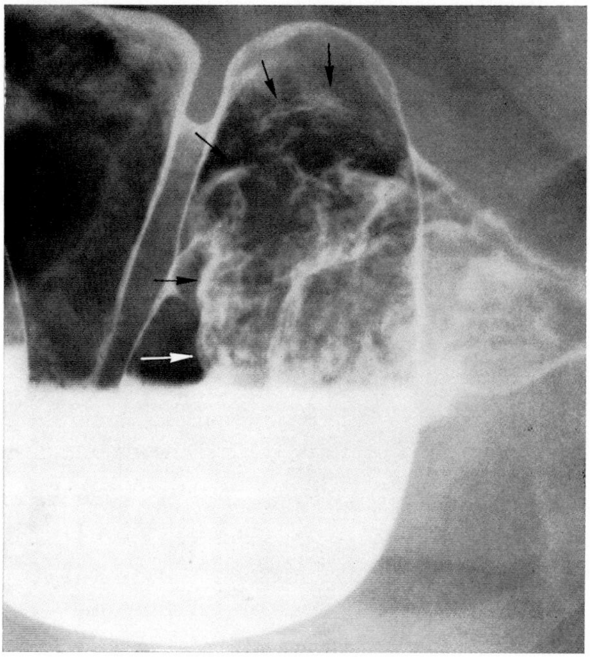

Fig. 51 c) In right recumbent position still in same position.

namely a sign of invasive growth, but even in the villous tumors it must be emphasized that the absence of the sign does not exclude malignancy. One should, however, always try to obtain profile views of these neoplasms (Figs. 48 and 50b).

Villous tumors are often accompanied by other neoplasms of the colon. Both adenocarciomas and adenomatous polyps have been diagnosed simultaneously, and in one of our cases there were two villous tumors, one situated in the middle part of the rectum and the other in the region between the rectum and the sigmoid.

Clinically as well as roentgenologically it is difficult to distinguish a villous papilloma from other lesions. Roentgenologically it is particularly the flat, wide neoplasms (Figs. 50a, b) that offer difficulties because they can be readily confused with local ulcerative colitis, and the smaller lesions can hardly be differentiated from polypoid carcinoma.

Unless the intestine is properly cleaned it might be difficult to distinguish large tumors from fecal matter, particularly if the tumors are situated in the rectum. In such cases roentgenograms with the patient supine and prone with the beam vertical and with the patient in the right and left lateral positions with the beam horizontal nearly always permit differentiation (Figs. 51a, b and c). This is because on change in posture the fecal matter changes in outline and position, while the appearance of the tumor does not.

8 Diverticular Disease

Introduction

Diverticular disease is a term introduced by Rosser in 1953. It includes colonic diverticulosis as well as diverticulitis and is employed particularly in the modern American literature as a general classification for both of these conditions. With an increasing population and longevity, this entity has become an important geriatric problem. Today the disease presents considerable therapeutic problems. The advent of more effective intestinal sterilization and better surgical technique with resulting reduction in morbidity and mortality justifies re-evaluation of the indications for surgical intervention. The claims for improved roentgen diagnosis have thus become more urgent, especially since there is often a considerable discrepancy between the roentgen impressions of the presence of diverticulitis and the clinical findings. It would be a most valuable help to the clinician, if the roentgenologist could identify those patients in whom the process has produced signs of acute or chronic inflammatory changes.

History

According to Drueck (1926), the diverticula in the colon were first described by Channel in 1710. One of the earliest descriptions of a lesion that might have been diverticulitis is to be found in the 1793 edition of Matthew Baillie's "Morbid Anatomy".

The first detailed account of diverticula is attributed to Cruveilhier in 1842. He described small pisiform tumors, resembling dark-looking varices, arising between the longitudinal bands of the colon. He was also the first to imagine that these swellings might become inflamed and he noticed that fistulae between the sigmoid colon and the urinary bladder need not be associated with cancer. In 1853 Virchow gave an anatomic-pathologic description of divericula of the colon and introduced the term "peridiverticulitis".

Graser (1898) was the first to make any serious attempt to understand the anatomy and pathology of diverticula of the colon; he was also the first to draw attention to the potential danger of diverticula as well as to observe that inflammatory stenosis resembles narrowing of the lumen by tumor and that the roentgenograms of both conditions are practically identical. He produced experimental evidence of the close relation of diverticular formation to the blood vessels through the intestinal wall. This relationship was earlier confirmed by Edel (1894) and Hanseman (1896). Graser also postulated that venous stasis was an important factor in the pathogenesis of diverticula. He believed that an increase in pressure in the bowel was necessary. He attributed this to constipation.

In 1907 Mayo realized that diverticulosis when inflamed can cause considerable symptoms and severe complications.

According to Kühne, Le Wald (1914) was the first to publish a roentgenogram of a diverticulum and thereby paved the way for diagnosis of the condition *intra vitam*. Until that time only descriptions of postmortem findings had been available.

In 1916 Drummond published his classical paper. His demonstration of the blood vessels around the colon has generally been accepted.

In the last few decades this field has received much attention in the literature. Many experimental investigations have been performed to elucidate the pathogenesis and etiology; roentgen findings and the pathologic changes found in biopsy and necropsy specimens have been compared, and in recent years interpretation of the roentgenograms has been revised. Changes formerly thought to be secondary to an inflammatory process are now regarded as prediverticular. Thanks to experimental research and comparative anatomic, roentgenographic and physiologic investigations it is now widely assumed that an increased motor activity of non-hypertrophic or hypertrophic musculature of the intestine is of causal significance. Intrasigmoid pressure and degenerative changes of ageing are some of the most important pathogenetic factors in the production of the gross and roentgenologic changes with shortening, marked interhaustral indentations, narrowing of the affected part of the bowel and diverticula.

Frequency

Diverticular disease is common. It occurs with equal frequency in both sexes and is especially prominent in obese patients. The incidence increases as the general population grows older. Routine clinical examination has shown a frequency of 1–23 percent; roentgenography of 6–23 percent and autopsy of 5–30 percent (Schreiber 1965). According to Clements (1969), the frequency is 35 percent at 45 years of age; according to Bergeron and Hanley (1960) and Meier (1966), 60 percent at 60 years of age; according to Welch (1958), 67 percent at 85 years of age. McCune (1957) and Welch (1958) believe that 6,000,000 of the United States 60,000,000 inhabitants over 40 years of age have diverticular disease. They also postulate that 1,200,000 suffer from diverticulitis, requiring proper diagnosis and treatment. According to Wigh (1965), the incidence of diverticulitis in the general population has proved to be comparable to that of duodenal ulcers.

Torres (1953) reported that 19 percent of all of his patients with colonic diseases had diverticular disease. In 35 percent the diverticulosis was diagnosed roentgenographically. In 56 percent there were signs of diverticulitis and 9 percent had peridiverticulitis with abscess and fistula.

Köhler (1963), who examined a large roentgen material at some large hospitals in south Finland and in south Sweden (Malmö and Lund), found that the incidence of diverticulosis in south Finland was only one-third of that in a corresponding material from south Sweden. He assumed that a contributory reason might be racial, but differences in dietary habits, mobility, general way of life or some other factors may equally well account for the difference in incidences.

In 1965 Fenger described a series of 191 patients with diverticulitis. Sixty-one percent were treated conservatively, while the remaining 39 percent were operated upon because of acute perforations, peritonitis, acute intestinal obstruction, suspected cancer or chronic intractibility.

Diverticular disease is most common in the sigmoid flexure. The next segment in order of frequency is the descending colon. The sigmoid is involved in 95 percent (Horner 1958), and 90 percent of the operations for diverticulitis were performed on the sigmoid flexure.

According to Barboka (1958), in 1956 diverticulitis claimed 1,360 deaths in the U.S.A., i.e. a death-rate of only 0.8 person per 100,000 inhabitants. Bolsford (1969) alleged that in those patients who underwent an operation, the real mortality was 7.8 percent. The three major causes of death are sepsis from anatomic leaks, perforations with overwhelming infection or delayed surgical treatment.

The above figures suggest that the diverticular disease infrequently results in death, yet in terms of morbidity it constitutes a major medical problem.

The Distribution of Diverticula in the Colon

Diverticula occur in the entire colon except for the rectum, where the teniae spread to form a broad sheath and this coherent sheath of longitudinal musculature strengthens the wall. According to Weston (1959), however, some 10 diverticula in the rectum are on record. From the cecum to the rectosigmoid junction the longitudinal muscle is bundled into the three teniae and only few fibers are left in the intertenial spaces. No diverticula exist in the areas covered by the teniae. They occur in the intervening spaces – usually between the mesocolic and the antimesocolic teniae – where the wall of the haustral pouches is formed mainly by the circular muscular layer. The circular muscle of the colon is usually described as forming a continuous, homogenous sheath, but some investigators, such as Morson (1963), Fleischner (1964) and others, have microscopically demonstrated that the small circular bundles of muscle fibers are separated from each other by thin strands of connective tissue, through which vessels penetrate and where the diverticula are situated. Painter (1970) alleged that the circular muscle fibers form semicircular arcs. Each arc consists of a double layer of circular muscle and the thin investing layer of longitudinal muscle.

Since the intestine is shortened in acquired diverticular disease, the inner surface of the gut has a corrugated appearance. The wall in the furrows is sometimes thin and made up of the mucosa, connective tissue of the submucosa, a minimal amount of muscle and the serosa. It is from these furrows that most diverticula of the sigmoid originate.

According to Slack (1962), the exact site of origin of the diverticula around the circumference of the bowel has never been satisfactorily established, but they are usually described as being arranged in linear fashion, forming four rows along the edges of the teniae, mostly in the wall between the mesenteric and antimesenteric teniae. They seem to be in close association with the mesenteric borders, but, according to Buckstein (1953), diverticula may be present not only at the mesenteric attachment but also in other parts of the circumference and are not infrequently found to grow into the appendices epiploical. To explain this Beer (1904) assumed the presence of local areas of muscular weakness in regions of the intestine other than at the pathways of blood vessels at the mesenteric border.

Congenital and Acquired Diverticula

Diverticula of the colon may be congenital or acquired. Congenital diverticula are usually solitary. Most of them are situated in the cecum and ascending colon and occur as isolated outpocketings in the anterolateral border of the intestine. Solitary diverticula in the sigmoid colon are apparently infrequent. The true or congenital diverticula are receiving increasing clinical attention. According to Daniels and Wood (1960), true diverticula arise as outgrowths of the bowel wall during embryonal development of the hindgut. They are composed of all layers of the bowel wall and may subsequently become atrophic. They are not so common as false acquired diverticula.

According to Rosser (1955), the acquired type possesses certain distinguishing characteristics. It is acquired during life and represents a herniation of the mucosa and submucosa through the muscularis propria and is enveloped by the serosa as it protrudes outward. 95 percent of them are situated in the sigmoid, but they occur also in other parts of the colon and, though rarely, also in the appendix vermiformis.

The acquired forms are traction or pulsion diverticula. Traction diverticula are very rarely observed. The first case on the base of a calcified lymph gland was described by Andrén (1955).

Acquired diverticula are of three types, *viz.* intramural, ridge and saccular. Intramural diverticula occur, as the first roentgenologic change, as a very fine irregularity of the outline.

The ridge diverticula present as ridge-like elevations and represent a further stage in the development of diverticulosis. It is thus a further extension of the mucosa beyond the muscularis. These diverticula produce a spiky outline of the same general configuration, but the spikes are usually slightly taller, wider at the base and may balloon to a certain extent.

Saccular diverticula present as smooth rounded projections varying in size; they are usually much larger than ridge diverticula.

Diverticula in the Cecum

Diverticula in the cecum and proximal part of the descending colon are congenital or acquired. The former are usually solitary; the latter, multiple. Half of all cecal diverticula are situated in the anterior wall; according to Shapiro (1958), they are shorter and their neck is wider than diverticula in the rest of the intestinal segment.

It is a relatively rare condition, said to occur in 1.7 percent of all cases of diverticulosis. The first case of acute diverticulitis of the cecum was reported by Portier in 1912.

Diverticulitis of the right colon may occur at any age, but according to Andersson (1947) it is most common in patients under 40 years of age, while the corresponding age for left-sided diverticulitis is between 50 and 70 years (Shapiro). The sex distribution is roughly equal.

The most common symptoms in the acute cases are pain and tenderness on palpation in the right lower quadrant of the abdomen. The condition is often mistaken for appendicitis and it is therefore a surgical disease. In the more chronic cases the clinical picture often gives reason to suspect a neoplasm.

Roentgen examination is obviously contraindicated when the most probable diagnosis is appendicitis, and in the subacute and chronic cases the most significant differentiation is that between intramural, extramucosal mass – inflammatory or neoplastic – and a mucosal lesion. Careful study of the cecum, appendix and terminal ileum will usually give the correct diagnosis. In diverticulitis the mucosa is intact. See below in "Differentiation from Cancer", p. 63.

Diverticula of the Appendix Vermiformis

Diverticula in the vermiform appendix may be congenital or acquired. They are important because of the frequent association with acute or chronic inflammatory disease: in the acute cases because of the tendency to perforation of the appendix and in the chronic cases because of the relatively high incidence of peritoneal pseudomyxoma (Ochsner 1961). Acquired diverticula were first described by Kelynek 1893. In 1926 Spriggs and Marxer reported the first case diagnosed roentgenologically. Later Gilmore and Mahan (1940), Wilson (1950), Rabinowitch (1962) and de Roies (1968) described some cases. Diverticula in the appendix have also been accidentally found in Malmö (Fig. 52). It is generally assumed that increased intramural tension is the main cause of constriction, which produces accumulation of contents behind it with stimulation of muscular activity and hypertrophy – with incoordinated muscular activity.

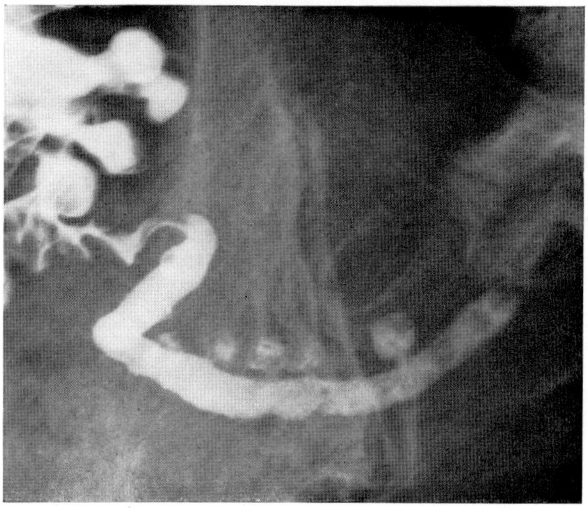

Fig. 52 ♀ 70 years. X-ray 9/1/70. Appendix with diverticula.

Pathogenesis of Diverticula

Much has been written about the pathogenesis of diverticula and their etiology, but neither are properly understood. There are, above all, three factors which must be regarded as dominant, namely muscle changes, weakness of the intestinal wall and the intraluminal pressure.

Muscular Changes

As early as 1910 Keith alleged that there is a strong contraction of the teniae in diverticulosis. He felt that this played a significant role in causing shortening, which throws the colon into circular folds. He also stressed that the circular muscle coat contracted irregularly.

Later investigators have also postulated that the primary factor in the diverticular disease is a change in the sigmoid musculature, and that this muscle abnormality precedes rather than follows the disease.

Thus Young (1965) wrote that the fundamental cause is probably local muscular thickening, which may exist without diverticula, revealed either in the films or in the specimens.

Williams, who in 1963 demonstrated that inflammation and contraction of the circular muscle contribute to the production of the changes in the roentgenograms, also wrote in 1965 that in diverticular disease the colon resembles a myostatic contracture. After having examined 80 specimens in the roentgenographic dissecting microscope and with a histologic technique to determine the pathologic anatomy, he argued that failure of the colon to elongate is the dominant mechanism in the development of the roentgenographic pattern.

The cause of the muscle abnormality is, according to some investigators, a spasm of the musculature in the sigmoid colon, while others believe that it is due to true hypertrophy, and, finally, some regard spasms in hypertrophic musculature as a possibility.

Among those who postulate that spasm was the main cause was Morson (1963). He found in his investigations of surgical specimens that the muscular abnormality was the most common and striking abnormality in diverticular disease. He thought that the muscle abnormality could be explained by the excessive shortening of the

bowel due to spasm. He felt that this view was strengthened by the absence of any detectable histologic abnormality of the muscle. He had not found any histopathologic evidence of hypertrophy.
Fleischner (1964) could not demonstrate evidence of muscular hypertrophy or hyperplasia in postmortem specimens. He thought that the gross shortening and narrowing of the colon were sufficient to explain the increase in the number and size of the muscle fibers in a given area. Like Williams, he suggested that the dominant lesion is a contracture of the longitudinal muscle.
Slack (1966) concluded after having made a careful study, particularly of the muscle nuclei, that the increased thickness of the intestinal wall in the diverticular disease is not due to muscular hypertrophy.
The assumption that there is no true hypertrophy of the intestinal musculature but only a spastic contraction is thus shared by many investigators, but some claim to have shown the occurrence of hypertrophy of the sigmoid musculature. To these belongs Arfwidsson (1964), who published extensive and careful histologic investigations of surgical specimens from patients with various types of diverticular disease. He found that the individual muscle cell nuclei in both the teniae and the circular muscle layer have a significantly lower density and are enlarged and that these nuclei are found less frequently; it may therefore be concluded – according to Arfwidsson – that thickened sigmoid musculature can be designated hypertrophy. He postulates, like Painter (1970), that the marked segmentation of the sigmoid lumen is a result of an increased motor activity of both the teniae and the circular muscle layer. Owing to contraction of the teniae the sigmoid colon is shortened and a partial segmentation of the intestinal lumen is achieved by the pleats formed in the entire intestinal wall. The colonic motor activity might thus play an important role in the pathogenesis of colonic diverticula.
Of those research workers who believe that it is a question of spasm in hypertrophic musculature, Edwards deserves mention because as early as 1939 he wrote that the most likely origin of diverticula was, among other things, hypertrophy of the circular muscle layer in the intestinal wall and that the roentgenograms exhibiting early stages of diverticulosis show irregular indentations between the haustra due to persistant tonic spasm of the circular muscle layer.
Celio (1952) had some confidence in Edwards' theory, but stated that such a hypertrophy is probably secondary to the spastic motor activity, caused by diverticulitis.
Finally, some authors have suggested that this roentgenographic pattern is due to fibrotic shortening of the bowel and is therefore an indication of previous diverticulosis (Goulard and Hampton 1954).
Summing up, it appears that most authors in this field are convinced that the intestinal musculature plays an important role in the development of the diverticular disease but no unanimity of opinion has been achieved as to whether it is a question of spasm, true hypertrophy or a combination of both.

Local Weakness

Another factor which might contribute to the development of diverticula is areas of weakness in the intestinal wall. Griffith (1961) has shown how vessels from the marginal artery of the colon pass round the outside of the bowel subserosally as far as the antimesenteric teniae and then become mucosal to join a rich vascular plexus, while shorter vessels run directly from the marginal artery through the wall of the bowel on either side of the mesenteric teniae to the submucosal plexus. According to Graser, these vessel passages, which contain both arteries and veins, constitute the weakest part of the intestinal wall. He showed in experiments that the sites of diverticula are closely related to the places where blood vessels pass through the intestinal wall. This relation was confirmed by Edwards as early as 1939. Also Slack (1960), Tagliacozzo and Virno (1961) showed by excellent anatomic dissection of operative specimens that the passages of the vessels through the sigmoid wall is the primary weak point.
According to Davies-Colly (1926), this weakness is due to the higher intraluminal pressure which forces the fatty tissue out along the vessel passages between the muscle fibers and thereby gives rise to areas of weakness. Bummer (1935) ascribed the weakness to an abnormal width of the vessel passages, and Oestern and Schreiber (1958) thought that it might be explained by a primary local disposition of the tissues with wide and numerous vessel passages together with

abundant loose perivascular fatty tissue that had undergone degeneration. Reifferscheid (1967) felt that the weakness was purely anatomical. The vessel passages, which in childhood and when relaxed run almost horizontally through the wall of the intestine, gradually assume an increasingly vertical course with increasing age and lack of tonus.

But there are many research workers who question the significance of the vessel passages. Buckstein (1953), for example, postulated that such a relationship of the origin of the diverticula of the colon to the sites, at which the bowel is perforated by mesenteric vessels, does not always hold. Fleischner (1964) was also unable to confirm the classical concept of a close relationship of diverticula and perforating vessels arteriographically. Tagliacozzo and Virno (1961), however, were able to explain the weakness by demonstrating such a relationship on the basis of their morphologic findings. When a diverticulum begins to develop the vessel is still within its canal. When the intraluminal pressure rises, the pressure is transmitted to the submucosal layer. The artery and its related loose connective tissue attachments push the mucosa into the gap and as the mucosa herniates outward, the artery is pushed away from the wall and comes to lie over the apex of the sac.

Some writers assume the existence of local areas of muscular weakness in regions of the intestine other than at the pathways of blood vessels at the mesenteric border. Many theories have been advanced to explain these weak points, among them, congenital, degenerative and inflammatory processes. But no theory has been universally accepted. Thus, Hartwell and Cecil (1910) like Pratt et al. (1942) thought that it was due to a congenital predisposition; Deelman (1957) to atrophy; and Lammonier and Martin (1957) to dystrophy; and Jordan and Boles (1960) to degenerative changes with a possible congenital origin.

Kühne (1958) claimed that the circulation of the blood through the intestinal wall decreases with advancing age with the result that the wall becomes less elastic and the contractions sluggish owing to insufficient contractility of the muscle fibers. Hence, diverticulosis is a manifestation of ageing changes in the intestinal wall with chronic hypoxemia of the muscle wall as a result. This opinion was shared by Boyd (1970). He wrote that the weakness seems to be due to the loss of tone and elasticity of the muscles, which is characteristic of the degenerative period of life, a view also held by Lockhart-Mummery and Hodgson (1931).

But Arfwidsson's histologic studies on surgical specimens from patients with diverticular disease refuted such theories. Neither were there any signs that "senile weakness" of the sigmoid wall was pronounced in older patients without diverticula. Thus, none of his findings seem to indicate that diverticula in the colon should arise as a result of weakness of the intestinal wall with advancing age.

Summing up, it is generally agreed that there is a good relationship between the origin of diverticula and local weakness. But opinions still differ widely on the cause and site of this weakness.

Increase in Intraluminal Pressure

It was realized as early as at the end of the 19th century that an increase in the intracolonic pressure was a strong contributory factor to diverticula. Thus, Zenker (1877) wrote that the main pathogenetic factor was intraluminal pressure and weak mural points. Graser (1898), Keith (1910) and Edwards (1939) also shared the opinion that the high intracolonic pressure was the primary cause.

Recent research has also demonstrated the occurrence of an increased intracolonic pressure, and as early as 1896 Hansemann showed experimentally that increased intracolonic pressure could induce hernialike protrusions of the mucosa. That increased intracolonic pressure does occur and that it can cause diverticula is accepted by most investigators, but not by all. Connel (1967), for instance, who performed comparative studies on the intracolonic pressure using balloons placed in the sigmoid colon, found in contrast to other investigators using catheters, only little difference between 19 controls and 25 patients with diverticular disease. He therefore thought that the diverticula might be the result of normal intracolonic pressure acting on a deficient musculature rather than of increased intracolonic pressure. Judging from the literature, his theory has not been accepted by any other author. On the contrary, both earlier and more recent investigators using multichannel manometric records have clearly shown the capacity of the sigmoid to withstand localized high pressures in a very short segment with areas only 7 to 10 cm away being unaffected. This is ascribed to the extreme narrowness of the lumen at this point and to the numerous prominent arc-like folds created by the thick bundles of the circular muscle, forced close together by the strong contraction of the teniae.

Formerly, constipation, straining during defecation and flatulence were often held responsible for the increased pressure. In 1953 Buckstein claimed that accumulation of feces and gas within the bowel was the most likely explanation, since fecal stagnation with hardening of the stool is apt to be greatest in the sigmoid.

Keith (1910) and Edwards (1934) proposed that increased spasticity of the intestinal wall may be contributory factors and also many modern research workers have arrived at the conclusion that the increase in pressure is due to increased motor activity. Arfwidsson (1964), for example, found with electromagnetic recordings a significant difference in pressure in the sigmoid colon in normal subjects and in patients with diverticular disease. The pressure was notably higher in the latter. He also found the frequency of strong waves to be significantly higher in diverticular disease. He therefore concluded that the marked segmentation of the sigmoid lumen is a result of the increased activity of both the teniae and the circular muscle layer. Owing to contraction of the teniae, the sigmoid is shortened and a partial segmentation of the intestinal lumen is achieved by the formed pleats, consisting of the whole sigmoid wall.

The sigmoid lumen is thereby radically diminished in size and some closed-off segments may be formed. In this way an extremely high pressure could be produced within the closed-off segments and herniation of the mucosa might occur via the available vessel passage of the sigmoid wall.

Painter (1964) and Reifferscheid (1967) also arrived at the same conclusion; the latter after simultaneous manometric and cineradiographic studies.

It may therefore be regarded as established that increases in pressure occur in the large intestine and that they contribute to the development of diverticula.

Symptoms

The symptoms of diverticular disease vary widely and sometimes the condition is asymptomatic. According to many investigators, as many as half of all cases produce no symptoms. Such patients may probably live without evidence of disability. In other cases there may be a varying degree of colonic disturbance with symptoms remarkably resembling those of irritable colon syndrome. It would appear, however, that the chances of developing symptoms increase with the duration of the disease.

The most common symptom is abdominal pain, which has been said to occur in 80 percent of all cases. It varies in severity and is usually situated in the left lower quadrant of the abdomen. Many patients report recurrent postprandial pain. Constipation is also common – it occurs in two-thirds of all cases, sometimes alternating with diarrhea. Changes in bowel habit, inability to effect easy and complete rectal evacuation, nausea, vomiting, fever, bloody stools, muscular rigidity and loss of weight have also been reported.

Because of the diversity of the existing symptoms McGregor (1958) suggests four stages:

1. Diverticulosis without symptoms.
2. Diverticulosis with symptoms.
3. Acute diverticulitis presenting a "left-sided appendicitis".
4. Chronic diverticulitis.

In the last group constipation with flatulence is extremely common. Defecation is incomplete. These chronic symptoms are accompanied by typical attacks of acute abdominal pain with vomiting, bladder trouble, meteorism and pain in the lower abdomen. Occasionally a lump can be palpated. The characteristics of the hyperplastic type of diverticulitis are obstinate symptoms of the type occurring in colonic stricture and the finding of a tumor.

Some authors believe that "the bleeding diverticulosis syndrome" should be classified as a separate clinical entity. Some also assume that superficially inflammatory erosions in the diverticula or in the colon can erode small adjacent arteries, while others think that the bleeding originates from an arteriosclerotic, inflamed or uninflamed vessel. It is, however, a serious complication and is generally observed as an intermittent minor bleeding, but the bleeding may also be massive and prolonged, especially in elderly patients with coexisting hypertensive and atheromatous cardiovascular disease. Without surgical intervention such cases will occasionally be fatal.

A major problem in the diagnosis of hemorrhage in diverticular disease lies in the fact that it can

be reached only by excluding other lesions. Therefore, rectal bleeding in the presence of diverticula always indicates careful roentgenography to find or exclude a polyp or carcinoma.
Since it is impossible to demonstrate a bleeding diverticulum by any direct test or examination, the diagnosis must be made by exclusion.

Roentgen Changes

The diagnosis of diverticular disease – at least in uncomplicated cases – is entirely roentgenologic.
According to Massik (1955), even anteroposterior scout films will often reveal collections of air – suggesting air-filled diverticula along the lower colon. The air-filled diverticula have a "bubbly" appearance, that of air in a slightly increased density interspersed with rounded spots of radiolucency. They are usually located in the left lower quadrant, most frequently in the pelvis, occasionally looking like a string of beads.
Fleischner (1967) also stressed the value of plain abdominal film. He claimed that a poorly outlined mass, surrounded by gas-filled bowel loops or obscuring of the standard fat-lines suggests a local inflammatory process, which indicates further investigation.
After the introduction of barium enema in 1914, this method was widely used.
However, it was soon realized that the mucosal relief method in this area too was better than earlier barium enemas and that in cases with numerous diverticula they could usually be seen more often in the postevacuation films than in the roentgenographs of the filled colon. This was partly because of the effect of superimposition of the filled colon but might be due also to the motor activity during evacuation, which caused previously unfilled diverticula to fill with barium.
During the last two decades it has been widely accepted that modern modifications of the double contrast method are better than others; firstly because they visualize diverticula that form no outline but are projected en face and, secondly, because they permit a better visualization of early changes.
As mentioned in an earlier section, most workers in this field agree that the primary change in diverticular disease is a change in the sigmoid musculature and like the pathologists, roentgenologists can distinguish four stages viz. the prediverticular stage, the diverticular stage, the inflammatory stage and complications.

Prediverticular Stage

The term was originally suggested by Spriggs and Marxer (1925). The roentgen changes are commonly seen in the sigmoid and often extending into the lower descending colon (Fig. 53). The normal segmentation is absent in the affected part of the colon. The haustrations are increased and irregularly spaced, and secondary smooth indentations appear. The transverse mucosal

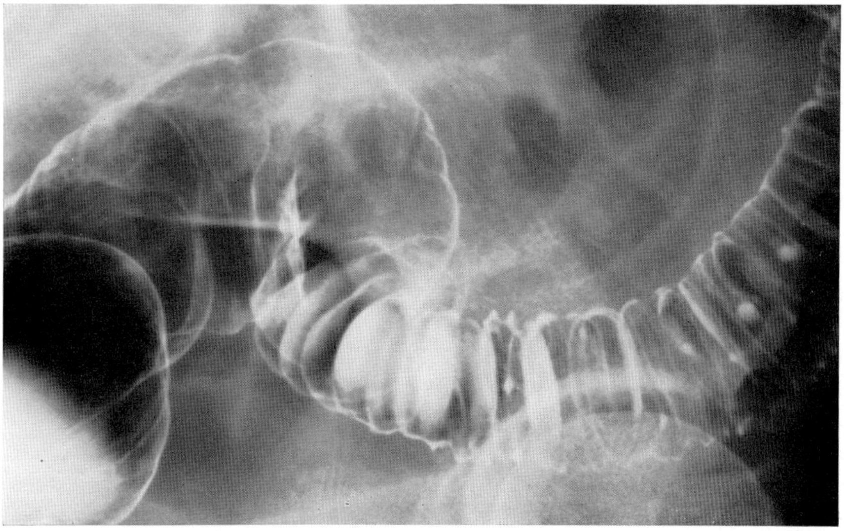

Fig. 53 ♂ 57 years. X-ray 10/2/70. Reduced lumen of the sigmoid. Increased parallel haustrations with some small spikes and specks.

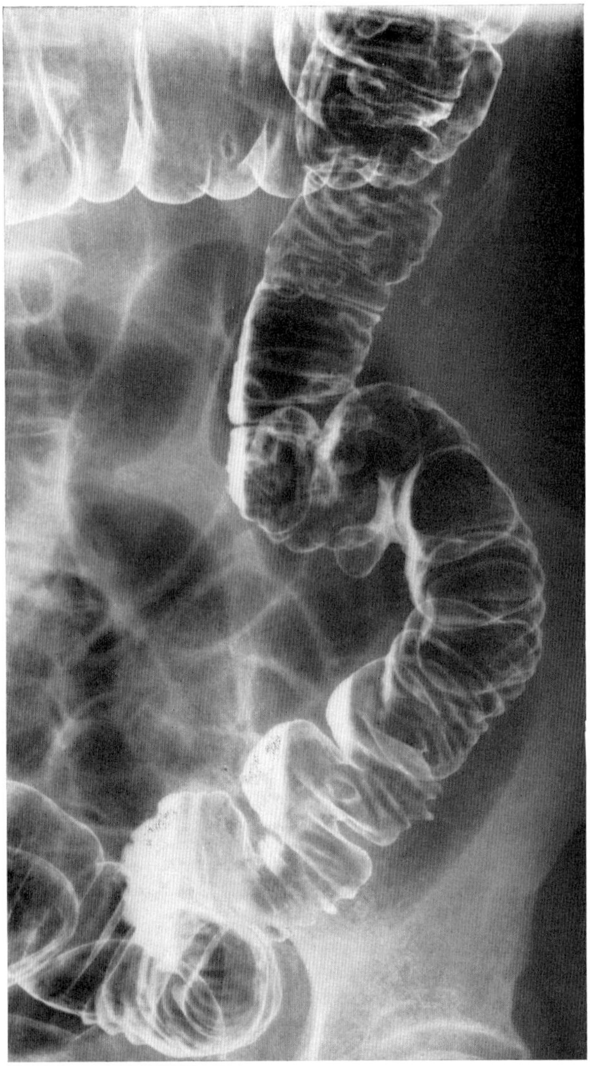

Fig. 54 ♀ 60 years. X-ray 26/1/70. The folds are more irregular.

folds are also increased in number and in size. They may be arranged like a palisade.
In other cases (Fig. 54) the folds are irregularly spaced and leave projections into the lumen of varying height. The spike seen in the roentgenogram is due to the remains of the lumen between two closely opposed inward folds. The margins of the bowel, which are usually narrowed and show lack of distention, appear grossly irregular with a serrated, ragged contour. The appearance of the sigmoid wall has been characterized as "concertina"-pleating and "ripple-border", but the mucosal pattern is intact.
With the use of the old barium enemas this type of pattern may disappear by the time filling is completed, and thus reveal the transient changes of an early and still reversible stage of functional bowel disease. At this stage it is thus a question of a spasm and colonic hyperactivity, in all respects similar to the irritable colon syndrome. In somewhat more advanced cases the above findings are fixed and more marked, and in such cases the sigmoid wall is constantly drawn together and the changes are due to actual thickening of the wall.
The pathoanatomic basis of these changes was for a long time a subject of controversy. The belief that the appearances were due to spasm as a result of inflammation can no longer be accepted, because there is no histopathological evidence of inflammation.
At this stage, according to Spriggs and Marxer, Arfwidsson and others, a large number of small intrusions of mucosa, resembling diverticula were demonstrated. They vary in size from a pinhead to that of a small pea and they are not manifestations of "prediverticular stage", but of established early diverticula.
Arfwidsson arrived at the same conclusion in his histologic study. He also showed that the lesions were situated close to a vessel.

Diverticular Stage

In addition to the changes in the prediverticular stage, diverticula can now be demonstrated in the roentgenographs. These are at first very small but after having passed through the muscular coat, they tend to broaden and become globular. They lie very close to the intestinal wall, and air surrounding contrast medium or fecal material in the diverticulum is common. The lumen of the bowel is narrowed and the haustrations are more irregular with smaller segmentations.
In tangential views the diverticula appear as outpocketings and in en face roentgenograms as rings (Fig. 55).
Pathoanatomic examinations show that the involved segment is narrowed and shortened and that the narrowing is now due to actual thickening of the wall. The margin of the bowel appears grossly irregular with deep undulating indentations, and the diverticula are frequently seen arising from the margin of haustral pouches.

Inflammatory Stage

Superficial inflammation in the diverticula is probably common, but it is usually self-limiting

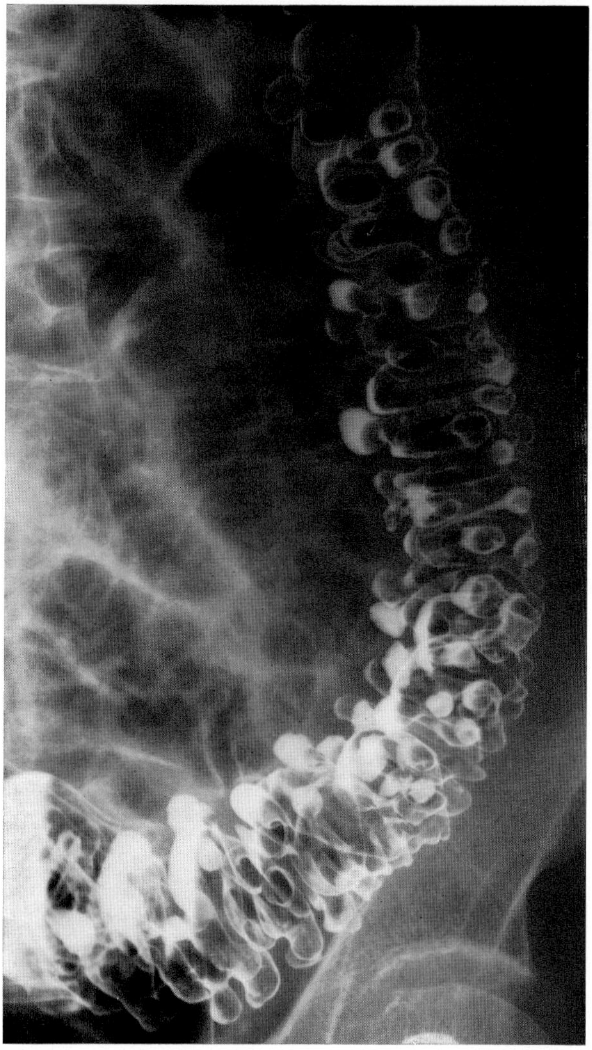

Fig. 55 ♀ 83 years. X-ray 10/2/70. Multiple diverticula, some in profile, some en face.

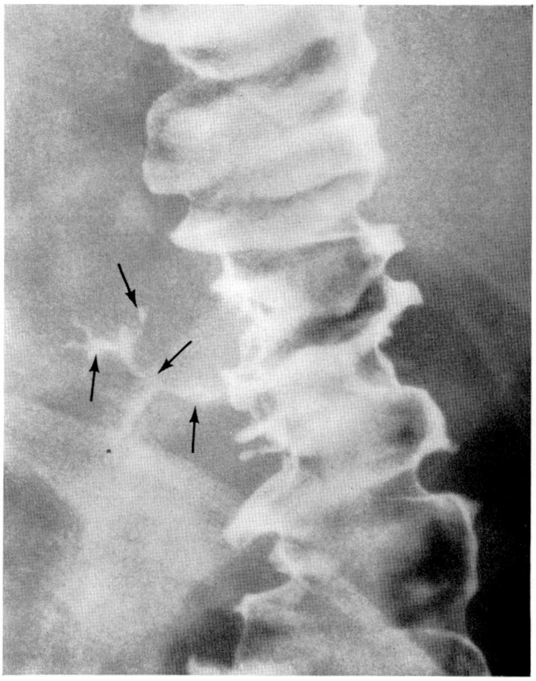

Fig. 56 ♂ 56 years. X-ray 4/7/63. Perforated diverticulum of descending colon. Peridiverticulitis.

and of no clinical significance. But sometimes the process does not heal, on the contrary, it continues. This is ascribed to a fecalith obstruction or hypertrophy of the wall at the neck of the diverticula resulting in suppuration, ulceration and necrosis of the sac, presumably due to mechanical or chemical injury from the retained fecal matter. The infection spreads through a microscopic or macroscopic perforation. The subsequent cellular infiltration of the wall causes thickening of the wall and narrowing of the lumen. Such an inflammatory swelling may lead to varying degrees of obstruction and according to the modern consensus of opinion it is not until such swelling and obstruction have occurred that it is possible to speak of diverticulitis.

The roentgen diagnosis of the inflammatory stage is to begin with very difficult, and it is sometimes impossible to distinguish between diverticulosis and diverticulitis. The diagnosis cannot be made before evidence has been produced of an extravasation of either minute or larger amounts of barium from one or multiple diverticula (Fig. 56). Local tenderness over a fluoroscopically demonstrated palpable tumor or ropelike thickened colon points to the same conclusion.

Other roentgenological signs of diverticulitis are local hyperirritability – the involved segment of the colon may be intolerant to barium, remaining filled and tending to empty rapidly – hypermotility, especially in the left colon, displacement of the coils of the small intestine upwards and away from the left iliac fossa by the inflammatory tumor mass, and rigidity of the involved bowel.

Sometimes there is a lengthwise spread of the infection between the muscular coats of the bowel or in the submucosal layers. This type is called intramural diverticulitis and offers different diagnostic and therapeutic difficulties. It is a striking anatomic variation from the one usually found in diverticulitis, because a longer segment of the bowel becomes involved in the inflammatory process.

Complications

The complications of diverticular disease are almost always of an inflammatory nature and they are usually secondary to the rupture of a diverticulum. They should be kept in mind whenever inflammatory masses develop in these regions in elderly patients with diverticulitis of the sigmoid.

Abscess and Fistula

Abscess formation and fistulous communication with neighboring organs are characteristic and fairly common complications of diverticulitis of the colon. Recurrent inflammation may cause the sigmoid colon to adhere to neighboring structures, and if a pericolic abscess forms, it may rupture into them with consequent formation of a fistula between the colonic lumen and another epithelial surface.

Hartwell and Cecil (1910) were among the first to describe such fistulization. According to Torres (1953) fistulization occurs in 9 percent, while others give figures ranging from 5 to 20 percent (Boles at the Lahey-clinic in Boston 5.1 percent, Hinton 5.1 percent and Feldman 15 percent). Sawyer found 20 percent of pericolic abscesses in his material, 8 percent of which were vesicocolic fistulae.

The diagnosis of gross perforation and formation of a paracolic abscess is readily made when the abscess communicates freely with the gut, but it is sometimes remarkably difficult to demonstrate the abnormal communications especially between different parts of the colon.

According to Wigh (1951), roentgenologically the peridiverticular abscesses are of two types: first, abscesses that are identified by a palpable mass contiguous with the bowel or by their displacement effect on the bowel; second, abscesses that are recognizable as such on the roentgenogram because their communication with the lumen of a diverticulum, which has perforated, is sufficiently large to permit introduction of an opaque medium.

Abscesses may develop upwards and downwards, anteriorly and posteriorly and may form adhesions and strictures of an ileal loop. But most abscesses fistulize.

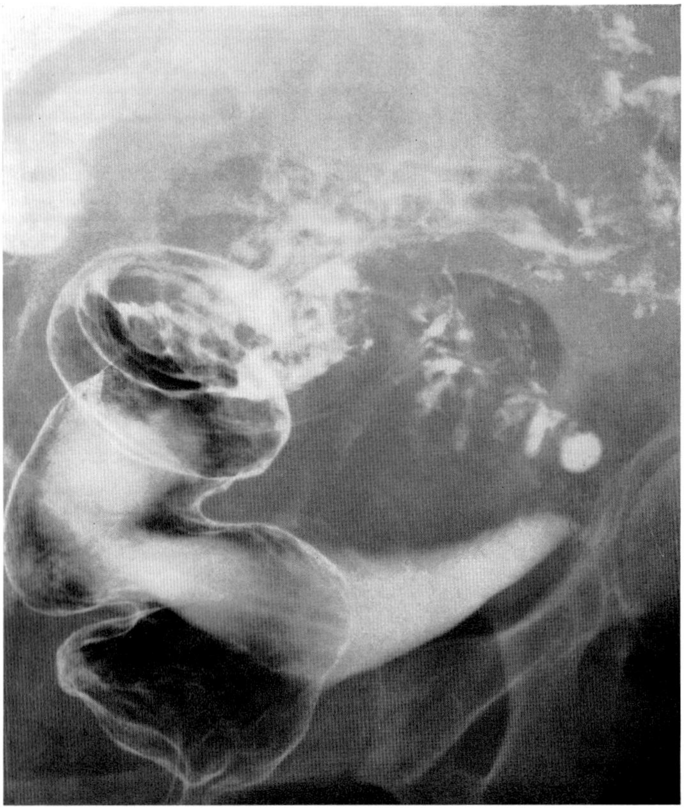

Fig. 57 ♀ 72 years. X-ray 4/6/58. Perforation of diverticulum in sigmoid with vesicocolic fistula.

Vesicocolic (Colovesical) Fistula

Vesicocolic fistulae are more common in men. They are rare in women, unless hysterectomy has removed the natural buffer between the colon and bladder. The uterus tends to keep the colon and bladder apart. The fistula results in urinary infection – cystitis is usual – and the passage of wind or even feces in the urine (Fig. 57).
Most non-traumatic colovesical fistulae in elderly patients are caused by rupture of a sigmoid diverticulum.

Colovaginal Fistula

The passage of air, feces or pus per vaginam are the presenting symptoms of fistulae, but the underlying pathology must be determined as such fistulae may be caused not only by diverticulosis – at least 30 percent – but also by a carcinoma of the bowel or of the uterine cervix or by irradiation.

Enterocolic Fistula

A pericolic abscess may rupture and thereby cause a fistula to form between the colon and adherent small gut and, rarely, the large bowel (Fig. 58). Intramural fistulae also occur, and their distance from the intestinal lumen determines if they are submucous or subserous.
Encroachment of a pericolic abscess upon the rectum is less common. A pararectal abscess may develop also in the retrorectal space. Such abscesses may rupture into the rectum and cause sigmoidorectal fistulae.

Colocutaneous Fistulae

Such fistulae may follow rupture of a pericolic abscess through the abdominal wall or the buttock via the ischiorectal space, but more often they are the result of surgical drainage of an abscess.

Retroperitoneal Extension

Perforation of a diverticulum of the descending colon, forming a fistulous tract or abscess, may clinically simulate a perinephric abscess and may be difficult to distinguish from other retroperitoneal lesions.

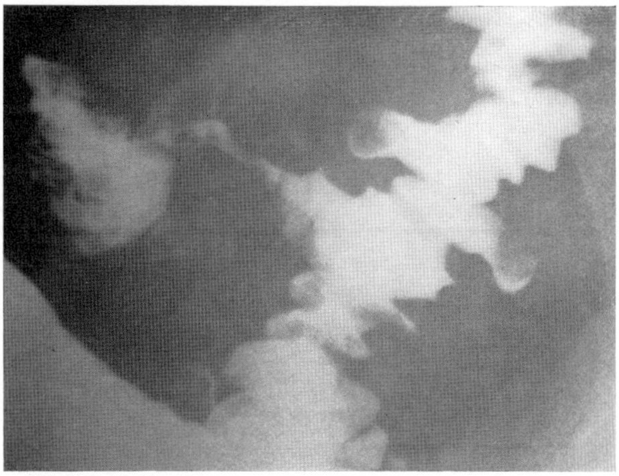

Fig. 58 ♂ 39 years. X-ray 10/1/65. Enterocolic fistula.

Stenosis

Obstruction by diverticulitis is relatively rare, but it may sometimes be so severe as to cause complete stenosis and even more frequent gaseous distention of both the large and the small bowel. Such patients are often referred to hospital suspected of subacute or acute ileus. If examined at all, we do not hesitate to examine these patients with the air contrast technique. We feel it safer to use air than a large amount of barium.
Fig. 59 shows such a case of stenosis due to diverticulosis in which the patient was later operated upon because of ileus.

Perforation

Diverticular perforation into the free peritoneal cavity is a rare complication. It may cause a severe septic peritonitis. The lesion is roentgenologically easily recognized with the aid of pneumoperitoneum.
Perforation is also said to occur occasionally after cleansing and diagnostic barium enemas. We have not seen any complication during the 20 years we have used this modification of the double contrast method in Malmö.

Differential Diagnosis

Irritable Colon

The irritable colon is an old clinical syndrome. According to Truelove and Reynell (1963), three clinical types can be distinguished, one in which

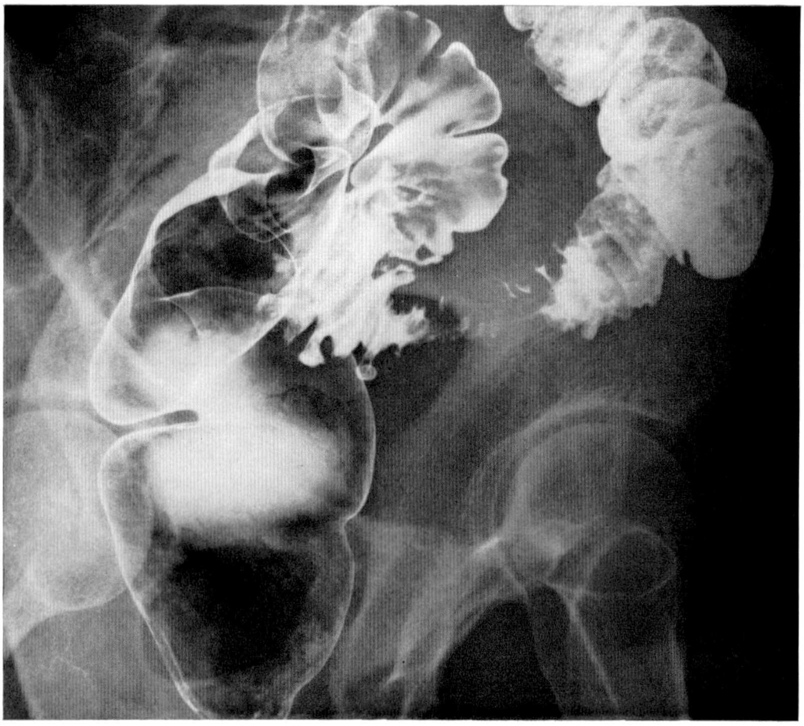

Fig. 59 ♂ 58 years. X-ray 10/8/60. Stenosis on basis of diverticular disease.

the clinical picture is dominated by diarrhea, lasting from a few hours to several weeks, one in which pain, usually in the left iliac fossa and of a continuous character with colicky exacerbations, and one in which the picture is dominated by pain with alternating diarrhea and constipation.

The roentgenologic changes of the irritable colon are, according to Golden (1936), well known. The sigmoid and the descending colon are abnormally narrow and the haustra are increased. The contrast medium rushes up rapidly to the splenic flexure. Fluoroscopy reveals repeated contractions, which are accompanied by considerable discomfort or even pain and the urge to defecate. Sometimes the irritability is so great that one is not able to fill the entire colon. Golden claims that it is a functional condition rather than an organic disease.

According to Lumsden, Chandhay and Truelove (1961), roentgenologically the irritable colon is largely diagnosed by the exclusion of organic lesions and demonstration of increased haustration and a segmental spasm. They thus arrived at the same roentgen criteria as Golden. They claim that these patients should not undergo any preparation before roentgen examination and that one should avoid all artificial irritation of the bowel during examination.

But the roentgen changes described by Lumsden, Chandhay, Truelove and Golden as typical of the irritable colon are also seen in the prediverticular stage of diverticular disease and it is at present impossible to make a roentgenological distinction between the two diseases.

Crohn's Disease

Differention from Crohn's disease usually offers no difficulties because the transverse stripes of contrast medium in Crohn's disease are straight and usually only about 1 cm long, besides which the mucosa shows inflammatory changes. In diverticular disease, however, owing to the projection of the stripes caused by the haustra or remains of haustra they appear somewhat curved and when the mucosa is examined in detail, no changes are noticeable.

A distinction between the two groups is of practical importance as postoperative complications are more common in patients with combined disease than after resection because of diverticulosis or its complications alone.

Ulcerative Colitis

Diverticulitis is rarely seen in association with ulcerative colitis. When it occurs it does so usually in persons in the third to fourth decades of life. The prognosis is gloomy. Complications are common and the operative mortality is said to be 15 times as high as that of diverticulitis alone.
Roentgenologic diagnosis requires demonstration of typical characteristics of both conditions, i.e. of diverticula and of ulcerations. The diagnosis is often not possible because only changes of one of the diseases are demonstrable. In early cases of ulcerative colitis roentgenography may show only the diverticula and in the chronic form the diverticula may be closed and the picture dominated by the changes of colitis. According to Beranbaum et al. (1965 and 1968), distorted irregular conical diverticula indicate inflammatory disease and should raise the suspicion of possible ulcerative colitis, even when ulcerations are not visualized. Sometimes the diverticular lesions may be predominant, sometimes those of ulcerative colitis.

Cancer

Differentiation between diverticulitis and carcinoma has received much attention in the literature. According to pathologists, coexisting diverticular disease exists in at least 10 percent of all cases of carcinoma of the colon. This figure is probably too low, since the diverticula are often considered unimportant in cases of cancer and are therefore not reported.
Clinically, it is often difficult to distinguish between the two diseases because the signs which differentiate them are not always demonstrable. The conditions also occur in the same age group (over 40 years) and both are localized mainly to the left side of the colon. Both produce bleeding. It is true that bleeding and loss of weight might occur more frequently in carcinoma, while abdominal pain, nausea, vomiting, chills, fever and urinary symptoms are in favor of diverticular disease, and that a smooth elongated tender mass favors the diagnosis of diverticulitis, particularly if it regresses with treatment, while a hard nodular mass suggests cancer. But it is often difficult, if not impossible, to make a firm differential diagnosis.
Roentgen examination is therefore necessary. Such an examination with the double contrast method will usually confirm the diagnosis, because with this technique it is possible to portray more mucosal details and detect diverticula, if any. It is today also possible to diagnose small polypoid carcinomas in the affected part of the intestine. Figs. 60a and b show such a case with

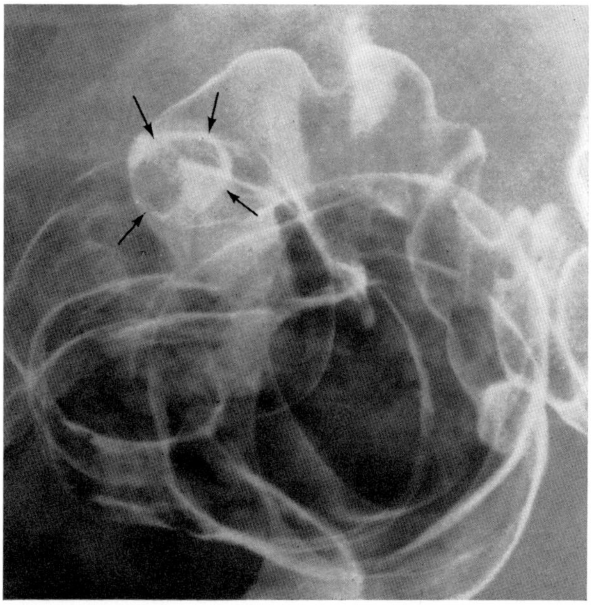

Fig. 60 ♂ 67 years:
a) X-ray 11/6/58. Sessile polyp, 11 mm in diameter, in affected part of Sigmoid.

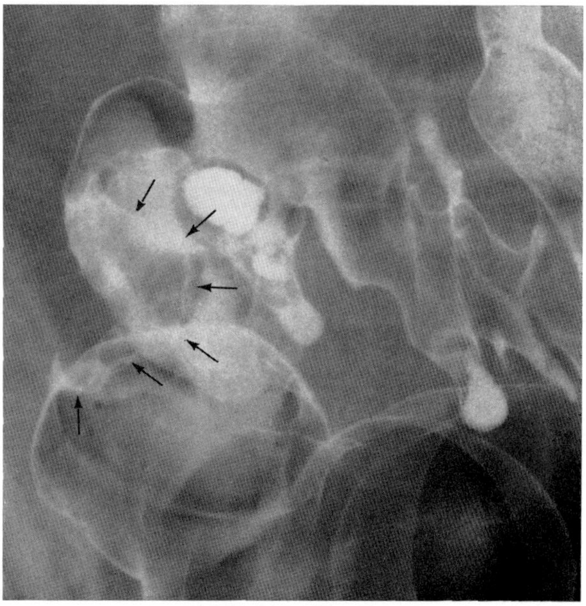

Fig. 60 b) X-ray 11/9/59. Now a carcinoma at the site of the polyp – 15 × 25 mm.

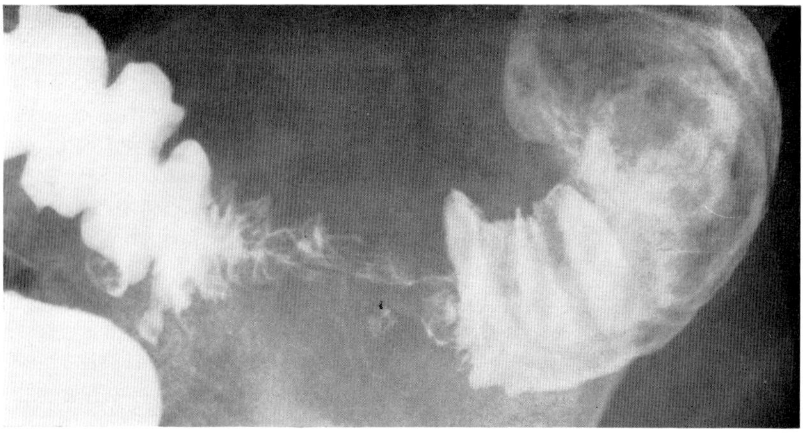

Fig. 61 ♂ 56 years. X-ray 154//66. Obstructing cancer with adjacent diverticula.

a polypoid tumor, adjacent to an area of diverticulitis. The follow-up examination one year later showed a typical carcinoma at the same site. The tumor had become much larger and had developed a typical indentation.

In some cases of chronic indurated or proliferative diverticulitis, where the fibrosis causes an irregular stricture and adjacent diverticula may become secondarily involved and obstructed, the differential diagnosis of an obstructing carcinoma may be raised (Fig. 61). It is often claimed that in such cases carcinoma has a shorter stenosis with a clear-cut shelf-like border at both ends and that the mucosa is destroyed, while the constriction is longer and the mucosa usually intact in the area of diverticular disease. Further, it is assumed that the presence of diverticula above, below and within the stenosed area favors diverticulitis, and since the induration in diverticulitis is inflammatory in nature and does not involve all the layers of the bowel wall, the resultant flattening or narrowing has not the complete rigidity and exact appearance of a malignant neoplastic process. Finally, a carcinoma will not improve with conservative therapy, while the spasm of constricting diverticulitis often will.

An abscess cavity may be due to a degenerating carcinoma in a patient with signs of diverticulitis, but this type of abscess is usually associated with a constriction caused by the tumor.

There are, however, cases where it is roentgenologically impossible to distinguish between the two diseases and where only the histological examination can exclude the presence of a sigmoid carcinoma. According to Colcock (1954), this was present in 16 percent of his cases of proven diverticulitis and in 4 percent of the patients with carcinoma.

In cases where it is difficult or impossible to differentiate between diverticulitis and carcinoma, the attitude recommended is one of surgical intervention in that there is much less danger in removing a portion of the colon for diverticulitis under the impression that it is a carcinoma than there is in leaving a carcinoma untreated because it is thought to be diverticulitis.

9 Crohn's Disease

Introduction

In 1932 Crohn, Günzburg and Oppenheimer were the first to describe an inflammatory condition of the terminal ileum, a condition now known in the United States as regional or granulomatous enteritis and in Europe as Crohn's disease. They underlined that this is a distinct clinical and pathological entity.
Colp (1934) described involvement of the cecum and colon by spread from the regional enteritis, and Musick (1936) described involvement of the pelvic colon by direct spread from the terminal ileum, the so-called "kissing" lesion.
As early as 1930 Bargen and Weber described a group of cases of colitis and emphasized the lack of involvement of the rectum and sigmoid. They called the condition "regional migratory ulcerative colitis". Eight years later, in 1938, Crohn and Berg called similar changes "right-sided localized ulcerative colitis".
Wells (1952) introduced the concept of Crohn's disease of the colon. It was soon realized that the colon might be involved not only over a short segment – segmental colitis – but, according to Brooke (1954), might also be much more diffusely involved. Crohn's disease of the colon is consequently now an established entity.

Course

Crohn's disease of the colon tends to begin in young adults or adolescents. Most patients present with symptoms in their late teens or early twenties, but the disease may appear for the first time in children or in early old age: the maximal incidence is in the third decade. Schofield (1967) has noted that colitis occurring in patients over 50 years was usually due to Crohn's disease of the colon. The usual age at onset of Crohn's disease of the colon has previously been shown to be markedly higher than that of ileal Crohn's disease.
Crohn's disease of the colon is usually chronic. It usually begins in the right half of the colon, particularly in the cecum. It is progressive and rarely disappears spontaneously. The course is more continuous than ulcerative colitis, in which the relapses, whether mild or severe, are often followed by long periods of complete remission and perfect health. Adequate medical treatment usually arrests the progress of Crohn's disease for a varying period, but not permanently. It is therefore suggested that the patient should be treated medically as long as possible. Surgery is often finally necessary for the majority of the patients. Crohn's disease is, however, a rather disappointing condition to treat surgically,though the immediate results of surgery are fairly good.
The symptomatic relief and improvement in general health after operation are often most gratifying and may endure for many years. But in 50 percent the disease will sooner or later recur, no matter which procedure is used. These depressing results have earlier served to dissuade surgeons from embarking on operative treatment, except for such complications as obstruction, persistent infection and prolonged disability.
The onset may sometimes be acute, though rarely. This is more common in ulcerative colitis. The acute cases of Crohn's disease of the colon are usually operated upon because of assumed acute appendicitis. A short segment of acutely inflamed ileum is the usual finding in this group of 10 to 40-year-old patients.

Clinical Symptoms

Many clinicians postulate that a reasonable diagnosis can be made preoperatively on clinical grounds. A careful history and knowledge of the appearance of the lesion in the earlier stages of the disease may clarify the diagnosis. The criteria are based on observations made in a large number of cases rather than on knowledge of the fundamental biological mechanism.

Diarrhea without gross bleeding is the most frequent complaint- sometimes the initial symptom. It is a true prolonged diarrhea with loose stools rather than the passage of blood and mucus with tenesmus, of which the patients with ulcerative colitis usually complain. It is often episodic, not so profuse and accompanied by an urgent desire to defecate.

The abdominal pain can be divided into three groups, depending upon the site, nature and radiation of pain:

1. Localized pain in the right iliac fossa, which often radiates through to the back, simulating urinary tract disease or rheumatic disorders.
2. Central abdominal pain, colicky and intermittent in nature, suggestive of subacute intestinal obstruction.
3. Upper abdominal pain, suggestive of peptic ulceration or gallbladder disease.

Loss of appetite and loss of weight occur early and seem to be constant.

Other symptoms and signs are chronic illness, vomiting, palpable mass, anemia, abdominal tenderness, abdominal distension, arthritis etc.

In some cases of Crohn's disease of the colon in an acute or subacute phase the lesions may lead to a severe hemorrhage, sometimes requiring colectomy.

Pathology

The etiology of the condition is unknown. It is not known whether the disease is a reaction to a specific etiological agent or whether it represents a limited number of ways in which the alimentary tract can react to a large number of etiological agents. This is open to debate, but it is undoubtedly true that this type of pathological process in the colon is being increasingly recognized.

Crohn's disease usually begins in the right half of the colon, particularly in the cecum. A predominantly right-sided involvement of the colon should always suggest the possibility of Crohn's disease. The rectum is always normal, even in the presence of severe disease of the anal canal, but is nearly always involved in ulcerative colitis. In the Malmö series all patients with Crohn's disease of the colon had changes in the terminal ileum. In Atwell's series (1965) the ileum was involved in 92 percent, and in Marshak and Lindner's series (1968) in 85 percent.

Crohn's disease is an inflammatory reaction, i.e. it is intramural, and involves all layers of the bowel, especially the submucosa. This involvement of all layers results in a significant thickening of the bowel and a narrowing of the lumen.

The histopathology was accurately described for the first time by Hadfield (1939). Later Warren and Sommers (1948) and Lockhart-Mummery and Morson (1960) realized that the pathological changes in the colon were identical with those of ileal Crohn's disease.

The changes in the cecum occur early. Some authors claim that the disease begins simultaneously in the colon and the terminal ileum, as both areas are usually involved by the time of the first roentgen examination. The initial changes of the cecum are indirect spasm and *deformity*. The lumen of the cecum is decreased and shows no associated mucosal changes in the early stages. It is often also shortened. In early cases this local narrowing of the bowel is reversible. The deformity is due to swollen lymph nodes at the ileocecal junction in early cases and to inflammatory masses or abscesses or adherent loops in later stages. These indirect roentgen changes produced by regional enteritis are not pathognomonic, but awareness of their appearance and underlying cause leads to a prompt and accurate diagnosis.

The intrinsic changes of the cecum are due to direct extension of the inflammatory processes, fistulae or enlargement of the ileocecal valve.

According to Morson (1968), Crohn's disease begins in the mucosa and histopathologically the typical lesions are inflammatory granulomas, containing epitheloid cells. The granulomas are localized mainly to the submucosa and the muscularis. All layers of the bowel wall are soon involved and this results in a significant thickening and rigidity of the bowel wall. Accompanying sclerosing lymphangitis causes severe edema, particularly of the submucosa. This raises the mucosa and gives rise to transverse mucosal folds with more or less deep grooves between them.

Tiny, shallow cone-shaped ulcerations, a few millimeters in diameter, are also seen. These ulcerations are similar to the minute ulcers in the early stages of ulcerative colitis. Sometimes they involve extensive areas of the intestinal wall. These small ulcers are usually observed only for a short time in the course of the disease.

In later stages of this usually progressive disease, the ulcers may become larger and deeper. They may undermine the submucosa and the depth may be accentuated by the overhanging margins, composed of hyperplastic mucosa, infiltrated by inflammatory cells. The deepest ulcerations involve the transverse and descending colon.

"Collar-button" ulcers are not uncommon. They tend to coalesce and become linear. In advanced stages multiple parallel longitudinal ulcers are seen, intersected by the transverse grooves, fissures or ulcerations. Ross (1965) calls these lesions "rake" ulcers, because they give the impression that a rake has been drawn along the mucosal surface of the segment involved. Some authors have postulated that the longitudinal ulcers are pathognomonic of Crohn's disease, but such lesions are sometimes found also in ulcerative colitis.

Ulcerations localized to a few centimeters have been described, as well as a longitudinal ulceration involving only one wall of a segment. The bowel lumen in such a segment is not notably narrow, but as the ulcerations produce spasm and contraction, the opposite part of the bowel becomes pleated. A striking appearance of pseudodiverticula has been described. This asymmetric appearance contrasts with the symmetric involvement in ulcerative colitis. The pseudodiverticula are very characteristic of Crohn's disease. The only other disease in which pseudodiverticula have been observed is infarction of the bowel.

When the longitudinal ulcers are associated with transverse linear ulcerations, they may produce the characteristic cobblestone pattern. This appearance is caused by crowded inflammatory nodules interspersed between serpiginous ulcers. Once this stage is reached, the lesions do not often regress.

One of the striking features is the skip lesion, in which apparently normal areas of the bowel alternate with diseased areas. It is widely believed that the disease may be discontinuous along the length of the bowel and two or more segments may be affected simultaneously. The process also tends to be discontinuous around the circumference of the gut. Sometimes terminal ileitis may be associated with one or more skip areas in the colon. This discontinuity of the lesions gives the impression that during its development the process spares smaller or larger segments of the bowel, but in all cases followed from the early stages, in the Malmö material, we have found a continuous spread from the proximal part of the colon to the distal part. This raises the question whether the skip lesion should be regarded as local healing of the process. Further investigation with this examination method should presumably provide an answer to this question.

Stenotic segments and strictures are common. They vary in length and in most cases they are multiple only rarely being solitary. They are seen in early stages and are then reversible. In later stages, the changes are due to marked thickening of the wall, caused by fibrosis. The changes also tend to be discontinuous around the circumference of the gut, so that the one side may be normal and the opposite side abnormal. It is generally believed that when all the features of benign stricture are demonstrated, a carcinoma is unlikely, but in the presence of any deviation, especially overhanging edges, differentiation from a carcinoma may be impossible and exploration necessary. Carcinoma is, however, rare in patients with Crohn's disease.

In later stages of the disease the entire mucosa may be sloughed off because of diffuse ulcerations. In those cases in which the bowel is diffusely and symmetrically involved and in which no typical features of granulomatous disease are demonstrable, differentiation from ulcerative colitis may be impossible. Marked thickening of the bowel, secondary to intramural fibrotic changes is common.

According to Morson, three macroscopic features of the disease may be recognized, namely:

1. That which gives rise to strictures, which may be short or long, single or multiple.
2. That which predominantly produces ulcers in the mucous membrane. In its earliest form they present as "aphthoid" ulcers.
3. That which gives the classical cobblestone appearance of the affected mucosa.

Crohn's disease of the colon is thus an inflammatory reaction that involves all layers of the bowel wall. Brooke (1959) wrote that owing to its gross appearance this condition can often be distinguished from ulcerative colitis, in which the inflammatory changes remain superficial even for many years.

Roentgen Diagnosis

The roentgenologic changes develop simultaneously with the anatomopathological lesions, and progress of the disease is accompanied by deterioration of the patient's symptoms.
The roentgenological changes usually appear first in the terminal segment of the ileum. There is a pathological mucosal relief and narrowing. In the acute stage it may be due to edema or spasm; in the chronic stage, to fibrosis. Ulcerations are common, as are small defects caused by polypoid changes in the mucosa. There may also be dilatation, proximal to an obstruction. Ileal lesions were invariably found in the Malmö series. In no case were the lesions confined to the colon.
In patients where Crohn's disease is still limited to the terminal ileum even before the process has extended to the mucosa of the cecum, there may be distinct roentgen signs in the cecum. These consist on the one hand of a reversible state of contraction and, on the other, of an indentation of the medial wall of the cecum. This deformity is important and is occasionally the only roentgenologic colonic sign associated with Crohn's disease. This change in the outline of the cecum occurs early and may be seen one to four months after the onset of symptoms. It may be due to extrinsic pressure by swollen lymph nodes at the ileocecal junction in early stages and by inflammatory masses or abscesses or adherent loops in later stages (Figs. 62a and b).
When the lesion encroaches upon the colon it involves all layers of the wall. As mentioned in an earlier section, the sclerosing lymphangitis causes severe edema, especially of the submucosa. This raises the mucosa and results in the formation of coarse mucosal folds with transverse more or less deep grooves between them as

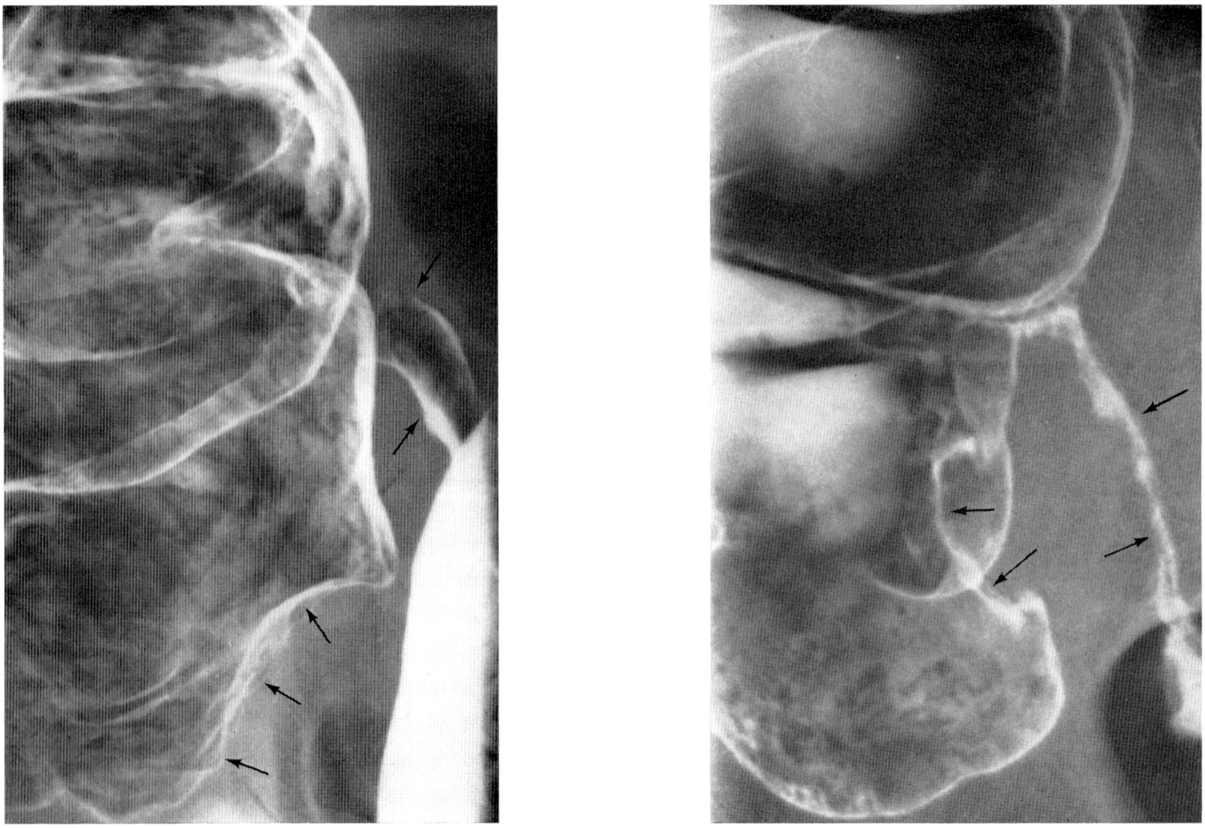

a b

Fig. 62 a) ♀ 35 years with *Crohn*'s disease. X-ray 4/2/59. Impression of lower medial part of the cecum and terminal ileitis.
b) ♂ 43 years with *Crohn*'s disease. X-ray 12/11/63. Impression of the upper medial part of cecum and terminal ileitis.

illustrated in Fig. 63. This reproduction shows also a swollen and inflamed mucosa with a longitudinal string of small ulcerations.
The most striking finding in a double contrast roentgenogram of early Crohn's disease is multiple transverse contrast stripes a few millimeters wide. They are more or less distinct. They are more than 1 cm long and are straight, while haustral remains, which are sometimes seen, are always curved. The contrast stripes must be caused by the contrast medium in the deep furrows between the mucosal folds, whether these are fiord-like fissures, true ulcers or simply folds (Fig. 64). These changes are reversible.
The mucosal relief is changed and often jagged. These spiky processes may be extensions of a

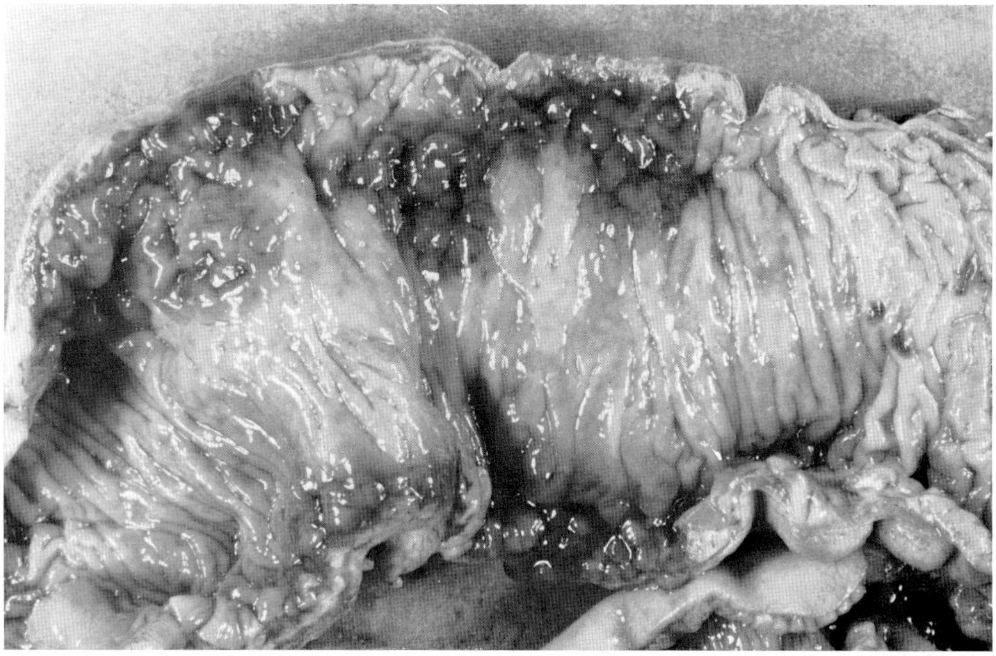

Fig. 63 Operative specimen of Crohn's disease. Significant edema with transverse folds and more or less deep grooves between them. Small ulcerations.

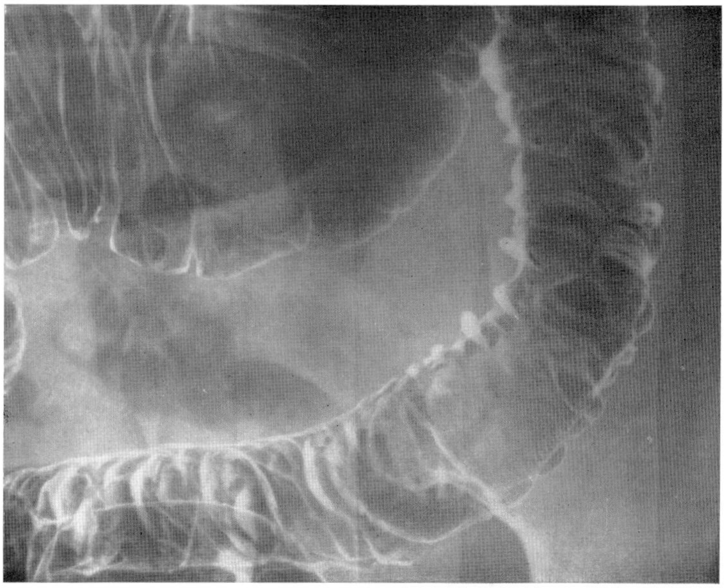

Fig. 64 ♀ 59 years with Crohn's disease. Follow-up:
a) X-ray 4/8/66. Multiple transverse contrast stripes and multiple ulcerations in the narrowed sigmoid and descending colon.

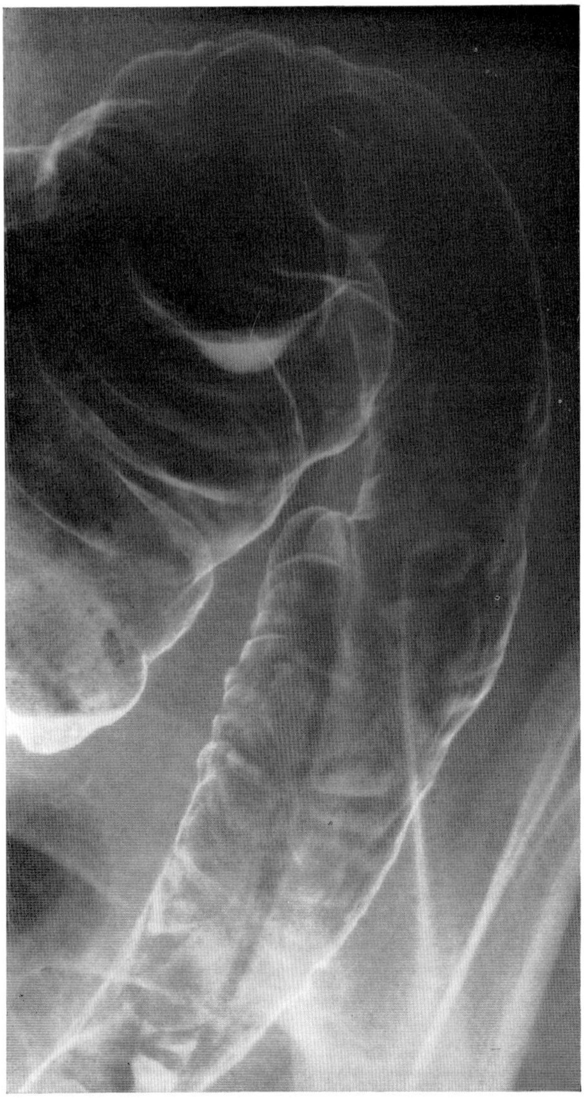

Fig. 64 b) X-ray 20/5/68. Control examination. Still transverse contrast stripes and narrowing, but no ulcerations.

transverse contrast stripe. As a rule, the spikes are so large that they must surely be caused by true ulcerations. They also vary in size and position. They can therefore not be grooves of the type described by Williams, which are smaller and according to Williams, due to enlarged Lieberkühn's crypts. Moreover, the haustra are often lacking and the intestinal lumen is narrower in the affected area.

As the disease progresses the ulcerations increase in number and become more hemorrhagic (Fig. 65). The image of the alternating mucosal folds and grooves is more distinct and the folds show numerous small aphthoid lesions, which the pathologists regard as probably the earliest macroscopic sign.

In Fig. 66 the inflammatory changes are still more advanced. The ulcerations are more numerous and more hemorrhagic. They also tend to coalesce to form longitudinal ulcerations and to branch in transverse direction. This reproduction also gives an impression of numerous transverse folds with deeper grooves between them.

A corresponding roentgenogram (Fig.67) showed not only the distinct transverse stripes, but also longitudinal stripes. On reviewing roentgenograms of patients with Crohn's disease we found these transverse stripes compatible with the appearance of the operative specimens in clinically mild early cases as well as in advanced cases.

Every roentgenologist who has worked with the double contrast method in this field has described the swollen mucosa and transverse ulcerations of Crohn's disease, but none have mentioned the diagnostic significance of these transverse stripes, caused not only by the ulcerations but also by the deep grooves or fiord-like fissures between the swollen folds. They are in fact so typical of Crohn's disease, that we at last have a pathognomonic roentgenographic sign of Crohn's disease, permitting differentiation from ulcerative colitis.

Another typical change in more advanced cases is, as mentioned previously, the development of innumerable closely-placed nodules between the serpiginous ulcers (Fig. 68). The changes are clearly seen in double contrast roentgenograms. They develop a cobblestone appearance. In such areas transverse contrast stripes are no longer seen.

Skip lesions, which occur in 15 percent of Atwell's material (1965) is another characteristic sign of Crohn's disease (Fig. 69). Areas of normal intestine occur between diseased segments of the colon. Two or more such areas are demonstrable. The length of such a skip area may vary from a few inches to several feet. The transition from the diseased to the normal intestine is fairly abrupt.

According to Bockus and many others (1965), the lesions in the colon are stationary and do not extend to adjacent intestinal segments. They state that they have never observed progressive extension of the disease distally from an intestinal lesion in the terminal ileum or proximal colon.

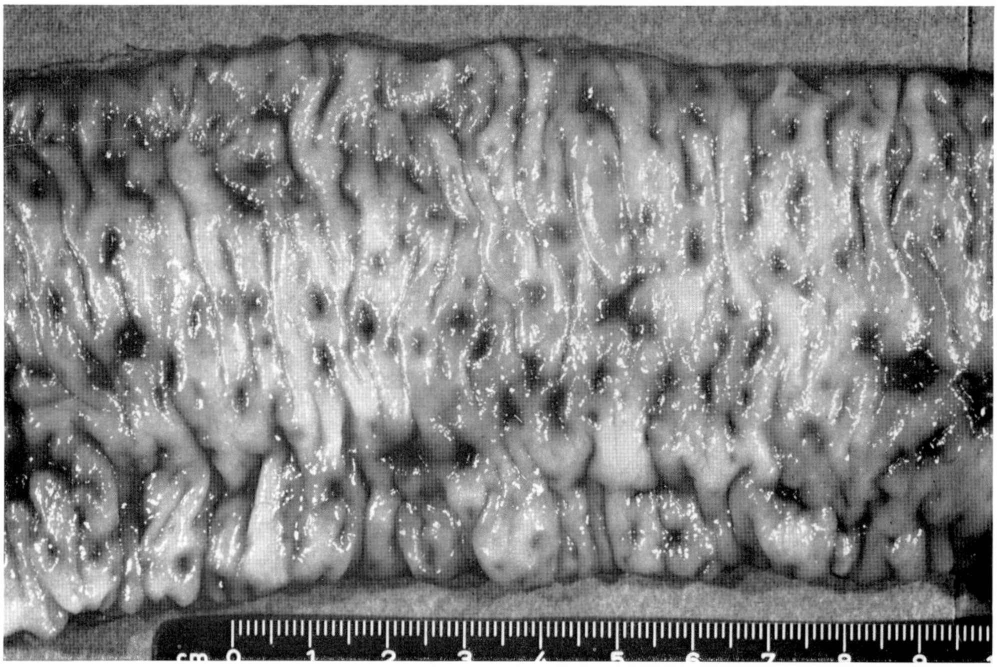

Fig. 65 Operative specimen of Crohn's disease. Inflammatory changes more advanced. More numerous and more hemorrhagic ulcerations. Aphthoid lesions on the edematous folds with deep intermediate grooves between them.

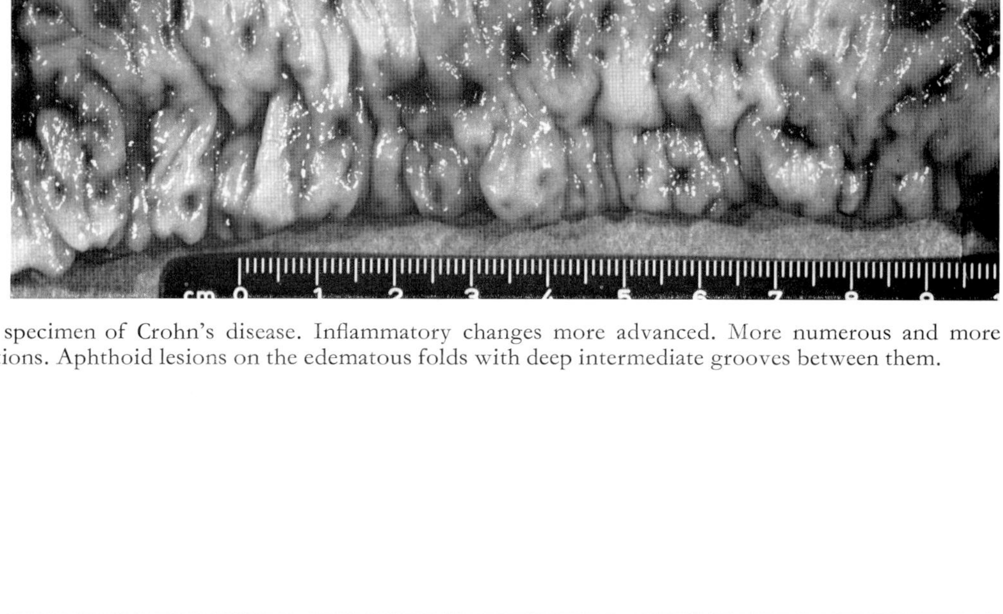

Fig. 66 Operative specimen of Crohn's disease. Still more advanced case. Now tendency of the ulcers to coalesce and form longitudinal stripes. Still numerous transverse folds with deep grooves in between them.

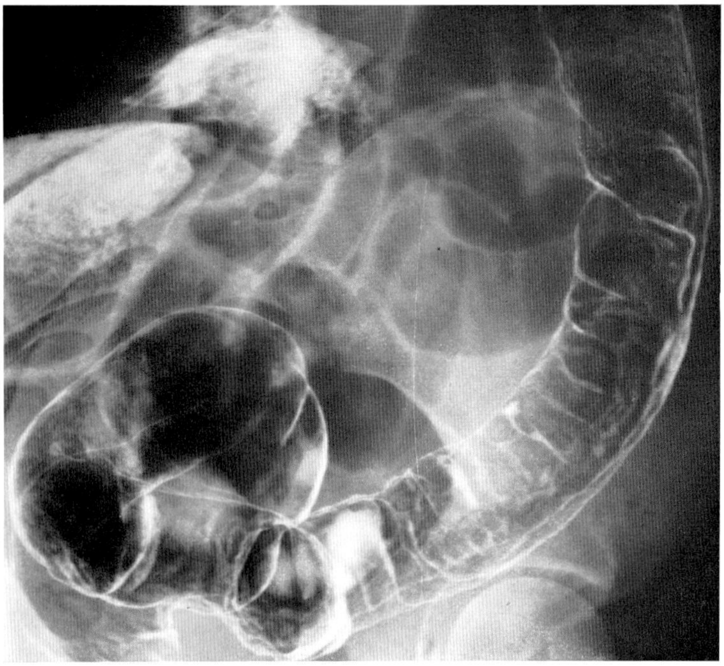

Fig. 67 ♀ 18 years with Crohn's disease. X-ray 31/3/64. Multiple transverse contrast stripes and longitudinal stripes.

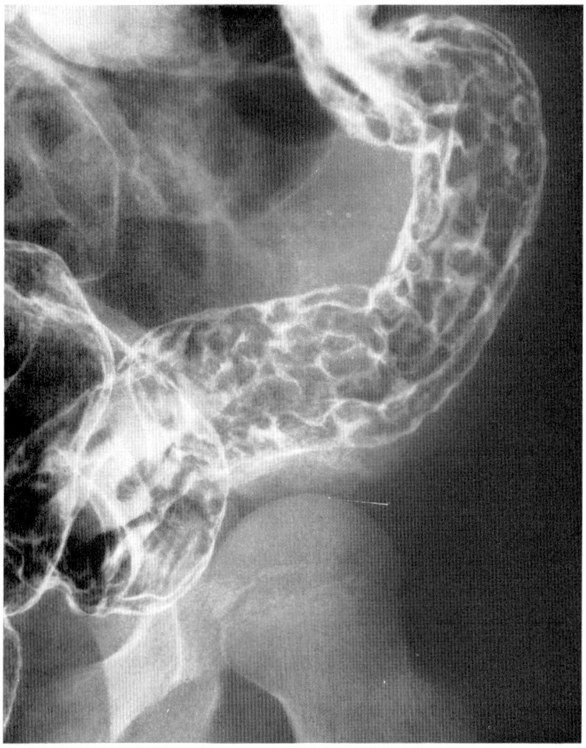

Fig. 68 ♂ 13 years with Crohn's disease. X-ray 7/3/70. Typical cobblestone pattern.

But the Malmö series contains many cases where the disease was followed with repeated x-ray examinations, in which it was possible to demonstrate that the process mitigates continuously distally (Fig. 70).

Complications

Abscess and Fistula

The ulcers sometimes develop into intramural abscesses, most frequently involving the transverse and descending parts of the colon. This may result in fistulization, as illustrated in Fig. 71. Owing to serous and peritoneal lesions, loops of diseased gut may become adherent to each other, to loops of normal bowel, to other viscera or to the anterior abdominal wall. If inflamed ulcers penetrate into the adjacent tissue a fistula is formed and may lead to intraabdominal changes.

Stenosis

Stenotic segments and strictures are common. They are caused either by a spastic contraction or by a typically increased thickness of the colonic

Fig. 69 ♀ 18 years with Crohn's disease. X-ray 19/9/63. Skip lesion. Deep impression in medial wall at junction between cecum and ascending colon. Normal mucous pattern of skip area of ascending colon. Cobblestone pattern in the narrowed hepatic flexure and transverse colon.

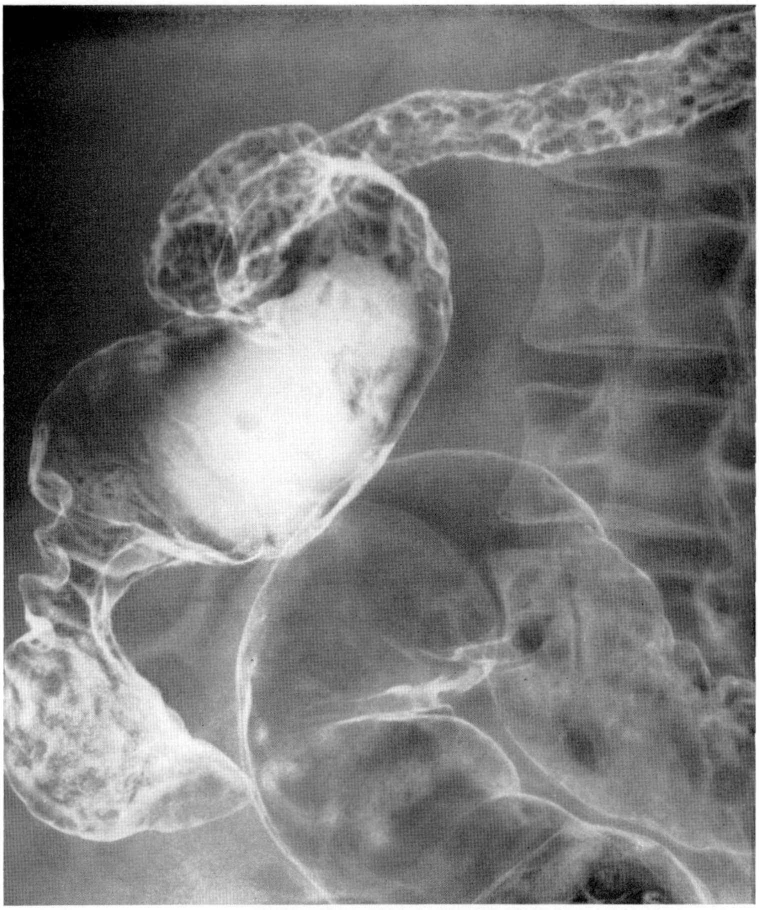

Fig. 70 ♂ 18 years with Crohn's disease. Follow-up:

a) X-ray 14/6/66. Impression of medial wall of cecum and multiple transverse contrast stripes in ascending colon – typical picture of Crohn's disease.

b) X-ray 26/8/66. After two months, treatment significant regression.

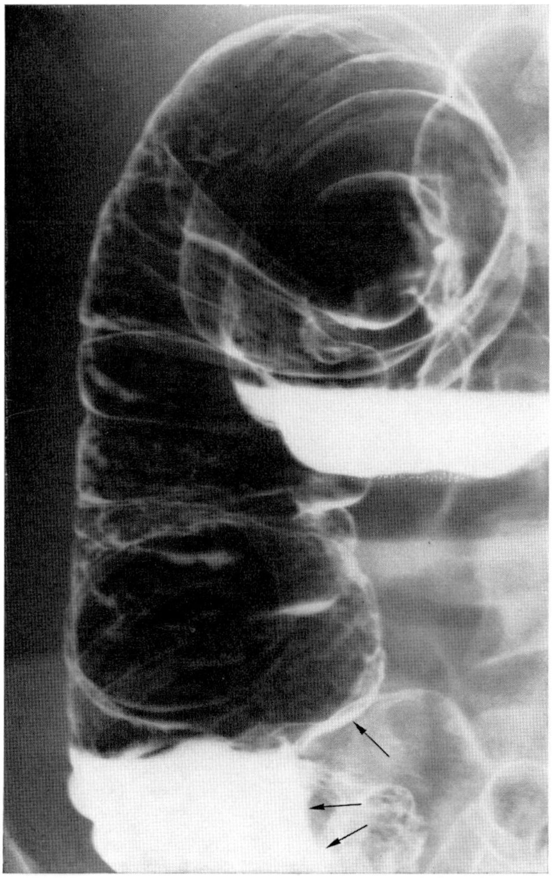

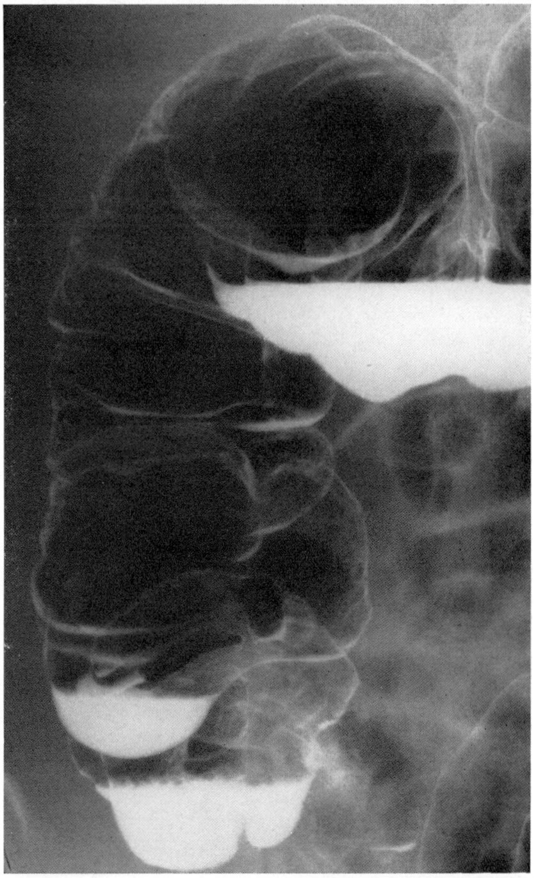

Fig. 70

a b

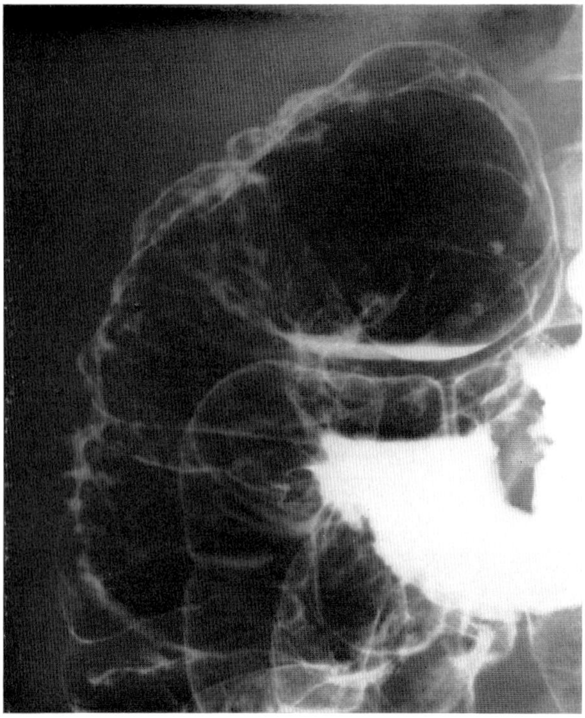

Fig. 70 c) X-ray 24/1/67. Progress of disease. Increased number of transverse contrast stripes and multiple ulcerations on lateral wall.

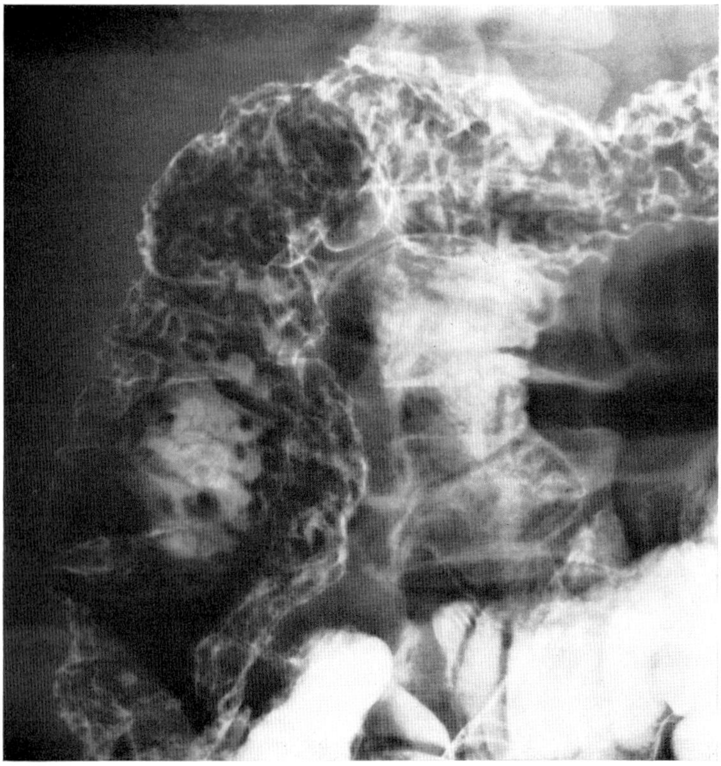

d) X-ray 31/3/67. Further progress despite treatment. Disease now involving not only ascending, but also transverse colon – cobblestone pattern.

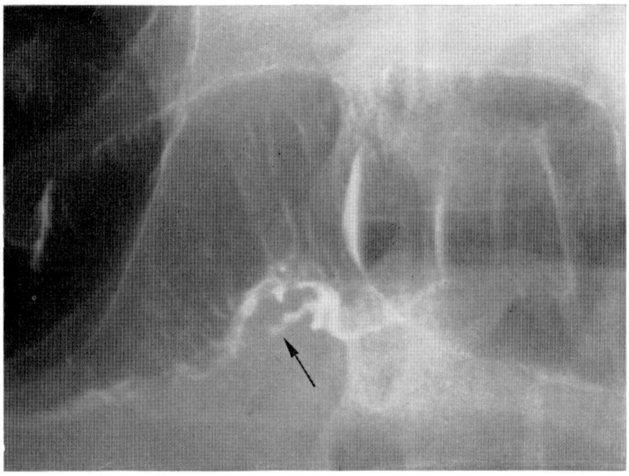

Fig. 71 ♂ 22 years with Crohn's disease. X-ray 7/5/68. Typical transverse contrast stripes in transverse colon with 1 cm long fistula.

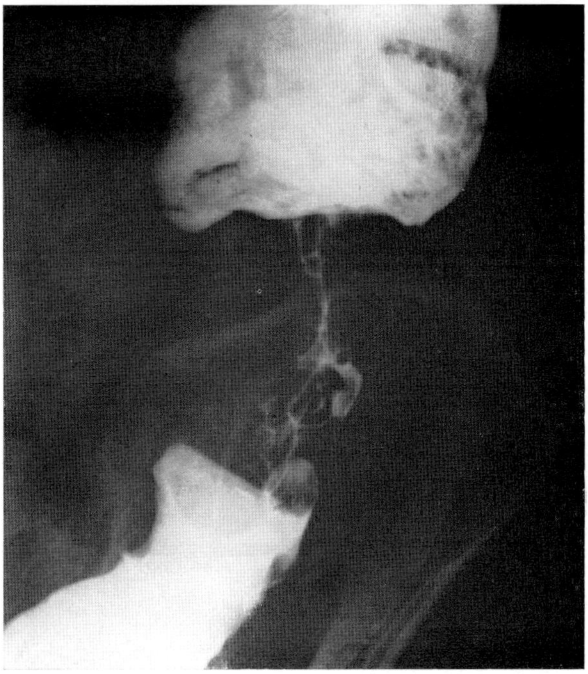

Fig. 72 ♀ 73 years with Crohn's disease. Advanced cuff-like stricture, leaving lumen, only a few millimeters wide and with irregular mucosal membrane.

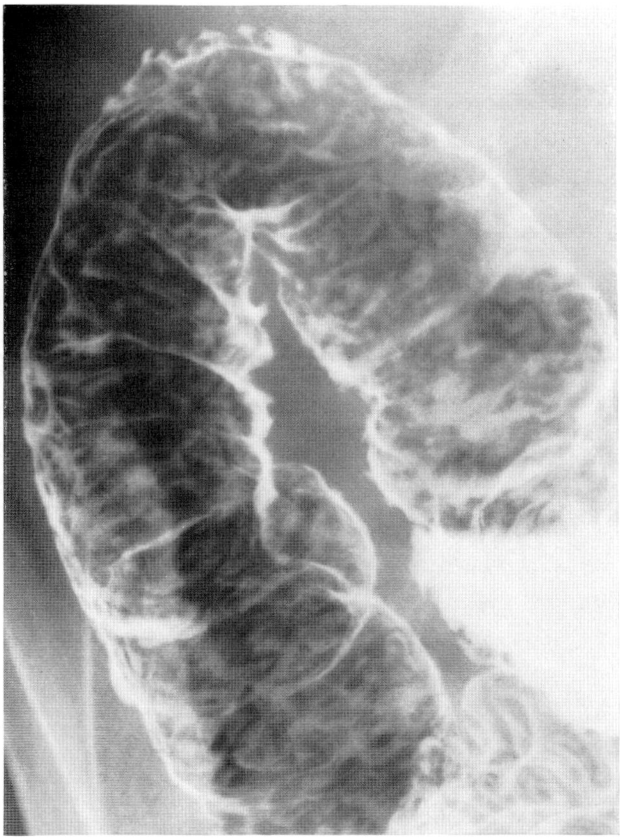

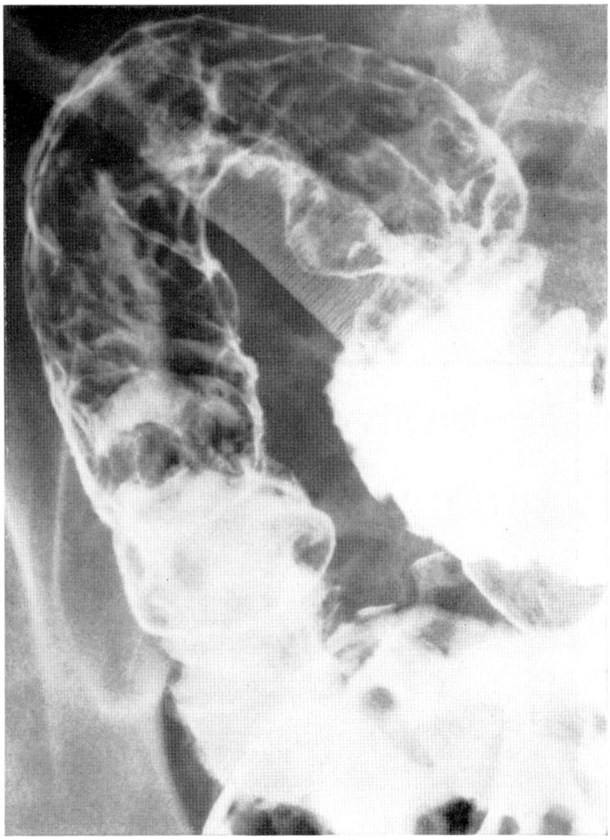

Fig. 73 ♂ 17 years. A follow-up case of Crohn's disease: a) X-ray 9/2/59. Multiple transverse contrast stripes, nodular mucosal pattern in cecum, ascending colon and hepatic flexure. Multiple ulcerations in hepatic flexure.

b) X-ray 2/4/59. Narrowing and shortening of affected part, nodular pattern remains, but no ulcerations and only few transverse contrast stripes.

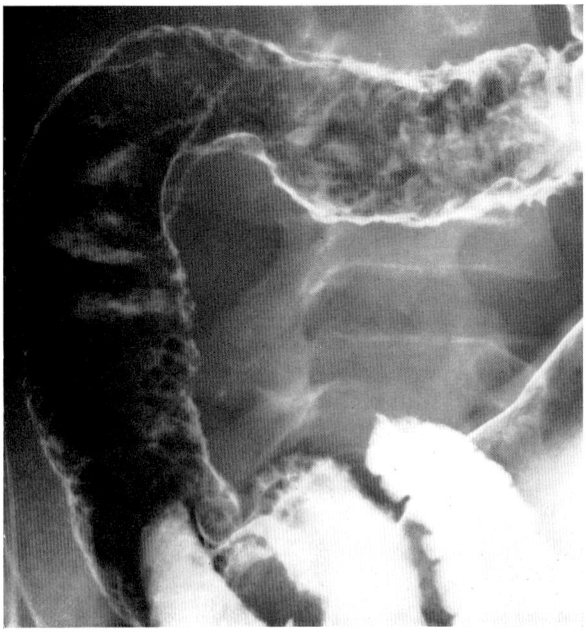

Fig. 73 c) X-ray 19/8/59. Less pronounced nodular pattern in cecum and ascending colon, but still a few transverse contrast stripes. Progress with ulcerations in transverse colon.

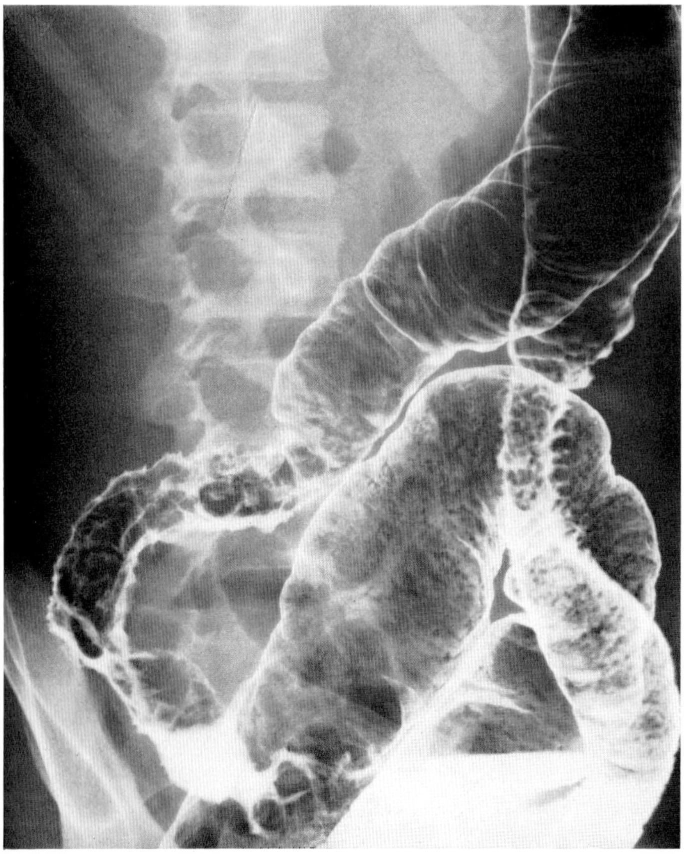

Fig. 73 d) X-ray 10/11/59. Significant progress of narrowing and shortening. Coarser nodular pattern with ulcerations in cecum, ascending and transverse colon. Now a nodular pattern with ulcerations and transverse contrast stripes in descending colon.

Fig. 73 e) X-ray 12/1/60. Further narrowing with a significant stricture in the ascending colon and more pronounced nodular pattern. Descending colon now quite normal.

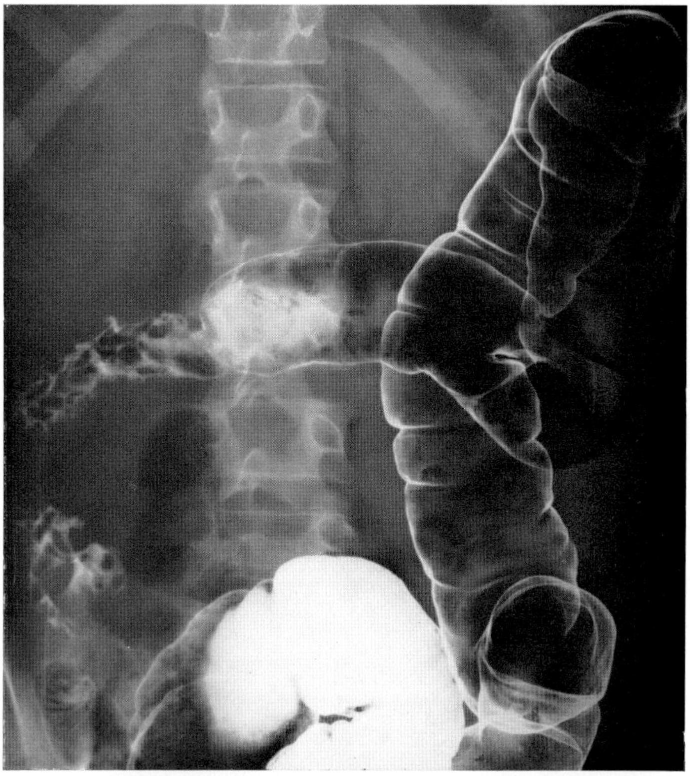

wall. In the earlier stages they are usually localized to the cecum. In later stages the stenosis is a common and typical change secondary to intramural fibrotic changes. If the stricture is eccentric and associated with an overhanging edge, differentiation from cancer may be impossible (Fig. 72).
The formation of a stricture may be relatively quick, as illustrated in Fig. 73.
After having passed watery stools for about one year the patient, a 17-year-old youth, sought medical advice. He was immediately referred for roentgen examination. Examination on 9 February 1959 (Fig. 73a) showed multiple transverse stripes in the cecum, ascending colon and hepatic flexure, a nodular mucosal relief and multiple ulcerations at the hepatic flexure. The lumen of the affected segment was also somewhat narrow.
On review two months later (Fig. 73b) the ulcerations had healed, but the mucosal changes in the cecum and ascending colon remained. Only a few transverse contrast stripes were seen. The degree of narrowing had increased since the previous examination.

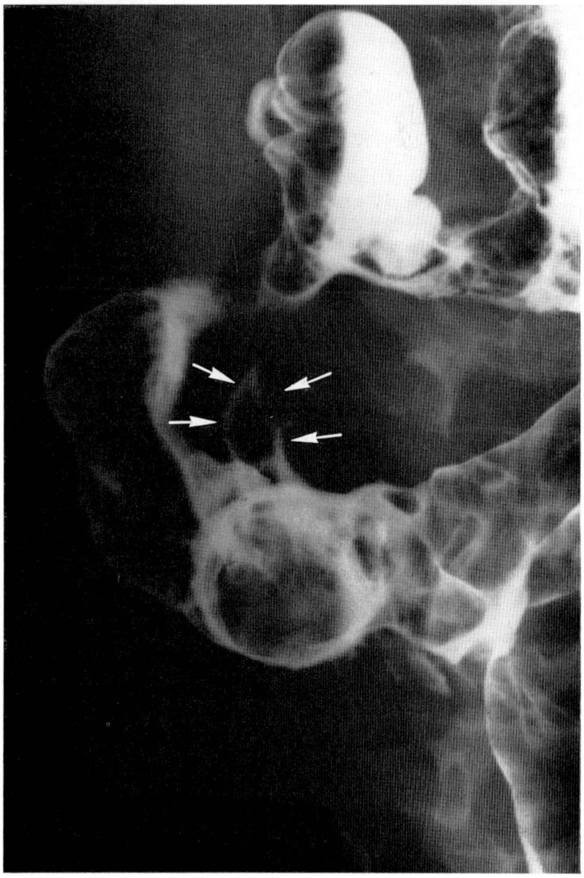

Fig. 73 f) X-ray 19/8/60. Again further narrowing and shortening. Now also fistulae from transverse colon.

Four months later, on 19 August 1959, the nodular pattern in the cecum and ascending colon was less pronounced but had progressed in the transverse colon, where ulcerations were also seen. A few contrast stripes were still present (Fig. 73c).
By the time of the examination in November 1959 (Fig. 73d) the cecum, ascending colon and hepatic flexure had shrunk considerably. The mucosal relief was still coarser and more irregular. Moreover, in the descending colon the mucosal relief was nodular with deep ulcerations and distally transverse stripes.
In the following two months (Fig. 73e) the changes in the descending colon had disappeared, while the shrinkage of the cecum, ascending colon and hepatic flexure had progressed and a severe stricture of the ascending colon had occurred. Those parts of the mucosa that could be judged were nodular as before.
At roentgen examination on 8 August 1960, i.e. about 18 months after the first examination the stenosis was more severe (Fig. 73f), the lumen was threadlike and a few fistulae extended from the affected part of the transverse colon.

Perforation

Free perforation into the peritoneal cavity must be rare. It was never seen in the Malmö series.

Toxic Dilatation

At one time it was believed that toxic dilatation of the colon does not occur in cases of Crohn's disease, but it does. Several such cases have been published in recent years. It is, however, much less common in Crohn's disease than in ulcerative colitis.

Anorectal Complications

Anorectal complications are very common in Crohn's disease, particularly when the sigmoid and rectum are involved. Many regard the presence of an anal lesion or a history that one had existed in the recent past as such a significant part of the clinical picture of Crohn's disease of the colon that its absence should arouse doubt concerning the accuracy of the clinical diagnosis. Lockhart-Mummery (1965) found such lesions in 80 percent, Cone in 68 percent and Appleman and Jackson (1962) in 36.2 percent.

Appleman classifies the lesions as follows:

1. Anorectal abscesses and fistulas.
2. Indolent anal or perianal ulcerations.
3. Extrarectal mass in the cul-de-sac or recto-vesical space.
4. Amoebic-like ulcerations of the bowel mucosa of the lower part of the intestine.
5. Granulomas of the rectum or the sigmoid usually indicating the site of an enterorectal or enterosigmoidal fistula.

The most common form is some ulceration of the anal canal, leading to one or more anal "fissures". They are seldom very painful and may be multiple. They are often broad and shallow and look indolent and undermined. Most are accompanied by marked edema, leading to soft tags around the anus. In some patients these ulcers of the anal canal extend out on the perianal skin, ischiorectal fat and the anal sphincters. Such ulcers and fistulae tend to extend forward to the vulva and groin.
These complications are an important aid in the clinical diagnosis of Crohn's disease and should be considered in the same light as the mucosal folds.
Anal complications may appear at any time in the course; they may sometimes be the initial complications. In some of these instances, there is nothing in the clinical appearance that suggests a specific cause. Therefore a roentgenologic interpretation of a localized lesion of the cloon in the presence of indolent anorectal disease should be tempered by clinical findings.

Differential Diagnosis

Brooke's and Cooke's Ileocolitis

The type of ileocolitis described by Brooke and Cooke (1951) is a primary small intestinal disease, which secondarily encroaches upon the colon. It causes large polypoid mucosal changes with stenosis and fistulization. Sometimes the roentgenologic changes are suggestive of Crohn's disease and sometimes of ulcerative colitis. Even operative specimens will not always permit a clear-cut differential diagnosis. Prévôt is of the opinion that Brooke-Cooke's ileocolitis might develop in both directions.

Ischemic Colitis

The acute onset of abdominal pain, alteration of bowel function and rectal bleeding in an elderly patient, especially with a history of signs of arteriosclerotic disease, should make the clinician consider the possibility of colonic ischemia.
The disease may be much more common than previously believed. Any portion of the colon may be affected, but it is most commonly the splenic flexure or the proximal sigmoid that is involved. The roentgenologic appearance of this disease varies with the degree and extent of bowel involvement. The roentgenogram is dominated by so-called "thumb print" indentations, originally described by Schwartz (1963). These are caused by submucosal hematomas and appear as oval or rounded masses along the walls of the rectum and sigmoid. Ulcerations vary in extent and depth, from superficial and multiple to single and deep or broad and flat. The changes also include irregular saw-tooth margins, polypoid protrusions and sacculations. The colon may be narrowed by spasm and submucosal hemorrhage and edema or by real strictures, which may be difficult or impossible to distinguish from cancer.
According to the literature, the changes sometimes resemble those in Crohn's disease. But the Malmö series of ischemic colitis included no case with transverse contrast stripes typical of Crohn's disease. On the other hand, ischemic proctocolitis may resemble ulcerative colitis roentgenologically, clinically and sigmoidoscopically, especially in the early stages.
The roentgenologic changes disappear in four to six weeks.

Ulcerative Colitis

The striking submucous edema in Crohn's disease of the colon causes such characteristic changes in the double contrast roentgenogram that the condition can be readily distinguished from ulcerative colitis, which is a superficial process of the mucosa. The mucosal folds with transverse stripes in the double contrast roentgenogram and the inflammatory mucosal changes are very characteristic and are not seen in ulcerative colitis. It was formerly claimed that the differential diagnostic signs of early Crohn's disease of the colon were confined to the right half of the colon and that the rectum was free, while the changes in the early stages of ulcerative colitis were most commonly found in the rectum and sigmoid. In younger patients with Crohn's disease the whole colon and rectum may, however, be affected from the very beginning. The lesions are always continuous.
It was also formerly assumed that the skip areas of involvement, longitudinal ulcers and cobblestone pattern were characteristic of Crohn's disease of the colon. It is true that these signs still facilitate the differential diagnosis, though the folds with the transverse stripes are the most important diagnostic sign.
The distinction between the two conditions is not only of theoretical but also of practical interest. Surgically, Crohn's disease of the colon often requires only a limited bowel resection as opposed to the disabling proctocolectomy necessary in extensive ulcerative colitis. The latter disease also carries a marked risk of development of malignant growths in the colon. Follow-up examinations must, therefore, be made of these patients at regular intervals.
Lockhart-Mummery and Morson claim that Crohn's disease of the colon and ulcerative colitis are entirely different conditions and that they cannot coexist. This view is being more and more widely accepted, but is in contrast to that of Yates and Crohn, who state that the two conditions may occur simultaneously in different parts of the colon.
Crohn reported this combination in 22 of 306 patients. We have also seen such cases in Malmö. Fig. 74 shows an operative specimen from a patient who was treated with colectomy. In the ascending colon there are coarse transverse folds and the transverse colon shows the nodular configuration of ulcerative colitis. After histologic examination of the operative specimen, the pathologist reported pronounced inflammation of the entire colon with an appearance consistent with Crohn's disease in the ascending colon and with ulcerative colitis in the transverse colon. This is exactly what was seen in the roentgenograms (Fig. 75). The transverse stripes of contrast medium in the ascending colon suggest Crohn's disease, while the changes in the transverse colon suggest ulcerative colitis. Our pathologist assigned this case to the group (5 percent of all cases) in which it is impossible to make a firm differential diagnosis between Crohn's disease, involving the colon, and ulcerative colitis, but the pathologic changes and the roentgenologic findings suggest that both were present.

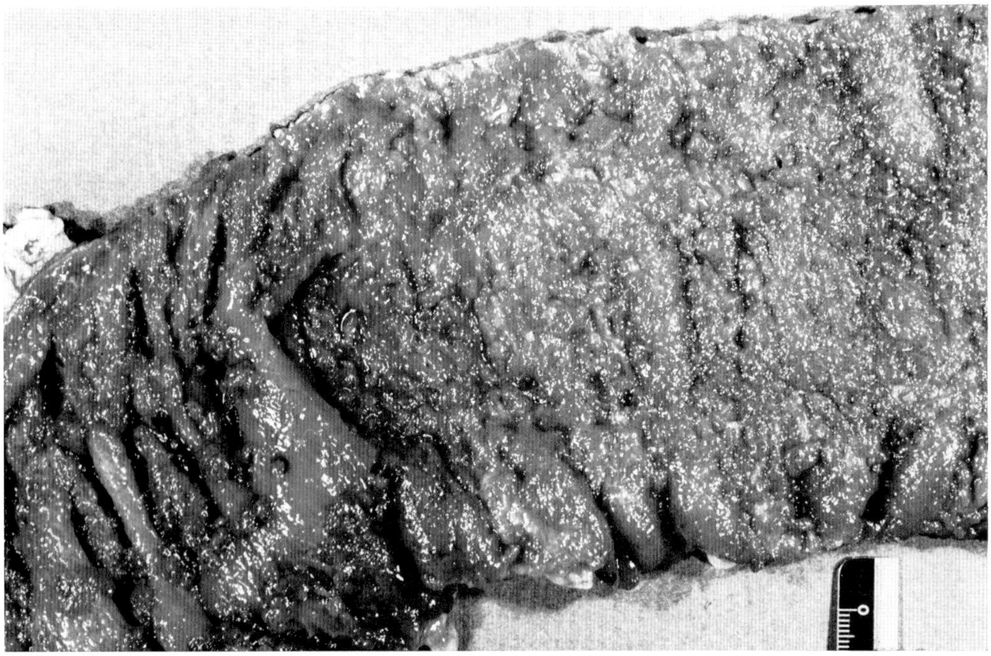

Fig. 74 Operative specimen from a patient with Crohn's disease in hepatic flexure and ulcerative colitis in transverse colon. To the left edematous mucous membrane with transverse folds and deep grooves – typical of Crohn's disease. To the right a fine granular pattern – indicating ulercative colitis. Histologically the same diagnosis.

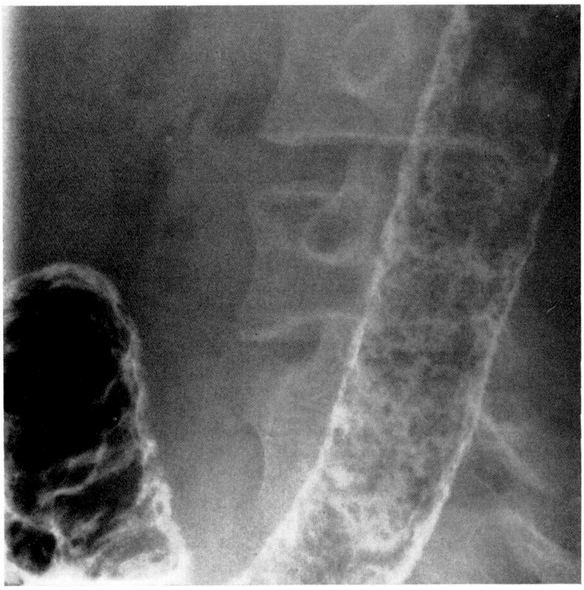

Fig. 75 ♂ 20 years. Same patient as in Fig. 74. X-ray 7/6/71. Multiple transverse contrast stripes in hepatic flexure, typical of Crohn's disease. Fine granular nodular pattern in transverse colon, indicating ulcerative colitis.

Tuberculous Colitis

Formerly it was difficult to distinguish Crohn's disease from tuberculous colitis, because both conditions produced similar pathologic-anatomic changes in the intestinal wall and both had a predilection for the ileocecal region. It was generally assumed that roentgenologic differentiation was possible only in advanced cases, while in early stages diagnosis required demonstration of tuberculosis of the lungs.

Today the situation is the opposite. In the early stages, when the process is superficial and both conditions show mucosal changes with small irregularities of the outline, a differential diagnosis is possible through the transverse contrast stripes so typical of Crohn's disease. In more advanced cases, however, the differential diagnosis is impossible (Fig. 76a, b). All layers of the wall are involved in both conditions. The rigidity of the wall increases and scar contraction develops. A constriction in tuberculous colitis cannot be differentiated from a deformity in Crohn's disease.

Cancer

Irregular stenotic segments and strictures are frequently seen in Crohn's disease of the colon. Such cases, especially if the mucosa is sloughed off because of diffuse ulcerations, are difficult to distinguish from cancer. However, it has generally been held in the past that there is no association between Crohn's disease of the colon

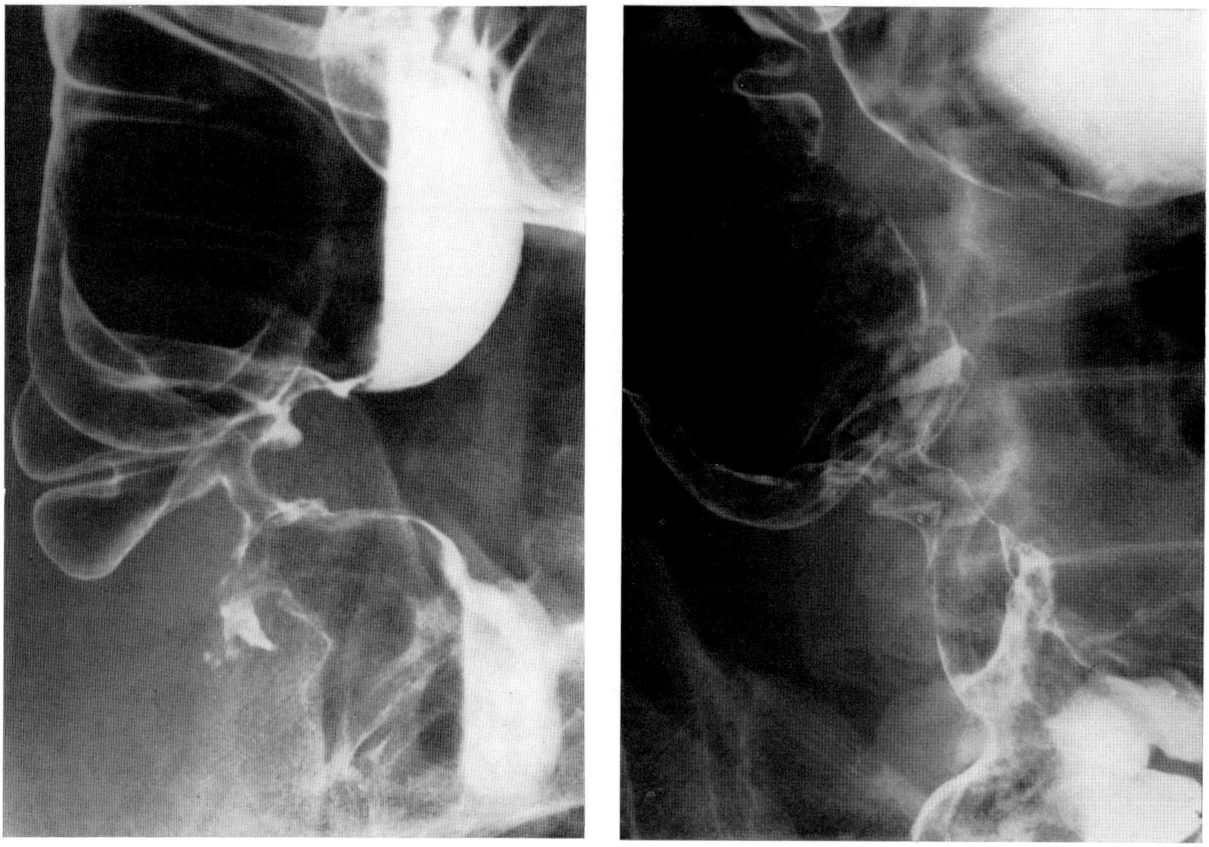

Fig. 76 a) ♂ 32 years. X-ray 21/4/55. Stricture and narrowing of cecum in case with tuberculous colitis.
b) ♂ 56 years. X-ray 8/8/58. Stricture and narrowing in case of Crohn's disease.

and carcinoma of the colon, although Perret (1968) found a frequency of 3.7 percent in his 82 patients. Since it is a considerably higher rate of cancer of the colon than would be found in a random sample of the population, he thought there might be some association between the two diseases. We have not found any such association in the Malmö material.

10 Ulcerative Colitis

Introduction

This is a rather violent and damaging chronic disease, characterized by remissions and exacerbations occurring at unpredictable intervals. It was first described as a clinical entity by Wilks and Moxon (1889) in their textbook of pathology. Cammeron and Rippman (1909) reported clinical findings, statistics and possibilities of treatment. The ulcerative stage of the disease was described by Smith in 1925.
Its roentgen features were described as early as 1912 by Stierlin. The first reference to its occurrence in children was by Jackman (1963).
Ulcerative colitis is relatively rare. It was formerly believed to occur with a frequency of approximately 25 per million inhabitants per year. It appears that both Crohn's disease of the colon and ulcerative colitis have increased in incidence in recent years. The etiology and hence the true nature of the disease is still a mystery.

Clinical Symptoms

The onset of the disease is often insidious and is ushered in by mild diarrhea and vague abdominal complaints, but is sometimes fairly acute with fever, abdominal pain and bloody diarrhea. Occasionally it is sudden with high fever, systemic toxicity, severe diarrhea and electrolytic depression or hemorrhage. This latter is an acute fulminating process of marked severity.
The cardinal symptoms are rectal bleeding and diarrhea; a toxic effect is often a prominent feature. The patients also often complain of abdominal pain. Less common symptoms are fever, loss of weight, vomiting or tenesmus. It should also be emphasized that distal proctitis may be associated with constipation. Sometimes, though rarely, a patient's main symptoms may be due to systematic complications of the disease.
Many investigators group their patients according to the clinical symptoms. One group of patients is characterized by violent water diarrhea, necessitating prolonged hospitalization, another by moderately severe symptoms in which the disease is confined to the sigmoid flexure and distal portion of the descending colon; a third is associated with terminal ileitis, and in the fourth, obstruction of the large bowel is the first sign of disease. Characteristic of ulcerative colitis are its exacerbations and remissions. These can also be obtained during appropriate and persistent treatment.
The disease is most common in elderly and middle-aged patients, but also occurs frequently in early childhood. In childhood the disease is apt to be more severe than later in life. Manifestations of chronic ulcerative colitis in children are the same as those in adults, except for growth retardation. Roentgenography of such patients will demonstrate the underdeveloped epiphyses of the bones.
In the geriatric population, the symptoms of ulcerative colitis are similar to those in the younger age group but are less impressive. The diagnosis is frequently delayed.
As mentioned above, the course may sometimes be fulminant. Some of these patients soon develop complications such as massive bleeding or perforation which may prove fatal, especially if surgical intervention is delayed.
Remissions may last for one year or even longer. But roentgenography during such periods will sometimes show continuous progression of the disease.
An analysis of the distribution according to the age at onset and to extent and severity of the disease revealed that more extensive and severe lesions developed in cases with early onset than

in those occurring later. The earlier the onset, the more marked were the subsequent changes.
All cases with involvement of the terminal ileum in addition to the large intestine, as well as the great majority of those with involvement of the whole large intestine, exhibited marked inflammatory changes in the bowel wall. Most of the cases with lesions confined to the distal parts of the large intestine or to the rectum alone showed moderate wall changes.
Summing up, the disease occurs most frequently in early and middle adult life but is not uncommon in early childhood. According to Lindner (1960) the ages at the time of onset were: first decade 2.3 percent, second to fourth decade 80.3 percent, fifth decade 9.7 percent and in patients over 50 years of age 6.4 percent.
The annual mortality rate is five per million inhabitants in Denmark and in the U.S.A. and Canada (1959). The disease shows no seasonal variations. In about half of all fatal cases the duration of the disease was one year or less, and in 35 percent, 6 months or less. The mortality rate increases steadily with the age of the patients. In 2 percent death was due to associated cancer of the colon.

Pathology

The pathology of ulcerative colitis was first described by Wilks and Moxon in 1875. It is a superficial mucosal inflammatory process and, in contrast to Crohn's disease of the colon, remains so for many years. The gross appearance of the bowel depends on the stage of the disease. The condition may originate anywhere in the large bowel, but in the beginning it is most frequently encountered in the rectum. It is generally accepted that the rectum is involved in more than 90 percent and that the inflammation spreads relentlessly proximally. It is not uncommon to find the left colon more often affected than the right. In advanced cases the entire colon may be involved (5 percent) and sometimes also the ileum. The most severe changes are generally seen in the rectum and in the descending colon. If the cecum and terminal portion of the ileum are affected, the appendix is also commonly involved.
It is generally believed that involvement of the ileum is due to retrograde extension of the disease into its terminal portion, which Crohn aptly describes as the "backwash" of the infected material. When involved, the mucosa is inflamed and somewhat granular with small shallow discrete ulcers and thus similar to those seen in the colon. They are always continuous with disease in the large bowel and are often associated with a rigid, dilated and incompetent ileocecal valve. According to Goligher (1954) ileitis is found in about 10 percent of specimens of patients subjected to colectomy because of ulcerative colitis but the extent of involvement varies from only a few inches to a foot and is only rarely longer. Involvement of the ileum may occur either early or late in the disease.
The initial gross pathological changes are those of a mild inflammatory reaction of the mucosa, usually in the rectum. The changes in this stage may be extremely sparse and include hyperemia, edema, and swelling of the mucosa, sometimes accompanied eventually by very small ulcers. The mucosa may bleed when swabbed; a sharp line of demarcation exists between the infected area and the normal bowel above. With the progression of the disease there will be a granular, hemorrhagic and smeared mucosa with a slimy, sanguinous exudate. The mucosa is deep red. In this early stage the bowel wall may appear to be slightly contracted owing to the edema of the submucosa and muscularis propria, but the outer coats are normal.
Ulceration is the predominant feature. It was earlier considered as a pathognomonic sign but it is not, since ulceration may be observed also in other diseases, which are ulcerative in character and have specific etiology.
The ulcers may occur early in the disease. The inflammatory process is then no longer localized to the mucosal surface but has penetrated deeper into the intestinal wall. At first the ulcers are very small. They are hazy, less symmetrical and less uniform than the so-called innominate grooves, which according to Williams (1965) are due to enlarged Lieberkühn's crypts. These are sharply defined and with a symmetrical, regular and uniform appearance.
If the process progresses, the ulcers become deeper and deeper. They may remain limited by the muscularis or they may penetrate through it, which will result in a deepening and widening of the ulcers, and sometimes also form a submucosal abscess with the "collar-stud" appearance. They often have a flattened base and overhanging margins.

If the ulcerations continue to increase in size, and especially in number, they have a tendency to coalesce. This may give rise to a continuous track of barium along the bowel contour and connected with the lumen at several points. Such a double contour varies in length from a few centimeters up to 30 cm.

The ulcerations may progress until only small islands of granular edematous mucosa remain between the ulcers, often extending deeply into the muscularis. As these islands are relatively raised up above the surface of the mucosa and project into the lumen, they may simulate polypoid lesions. Thus, in ulcerative colitis there may be both adenomatous polyps and pseudopolyps.

The adenomatous polyps observed in the Malmö material of ulcerative colitis were 4 times more common than expected. This may perhaps be explained by the assumption that colitis stimulates growth of an otherwise stationary latent adenoma. Another possibility is that the colitis, by some sort of autoimmunization, causes the adenoma.

The pseudopolyps are not polyps in the strict sense of the word. "Inflammatory polyp" would be a better description as it indicates the way in which these polyps are formed. The histologic appearance varies widely, but cellular infiltration, characteristic of ulcerative colitis, is a feature common to all. Some may be organized and composed of stratified inflammatory exudate. In such cases there is no mucosal lining. Others may be projections of mucosa with a core of connective tissue and a mucosal lining, possessing all characteristics observed in other areas of the diseased colon.

Inflammatory polyps are found most frequently in the rectum, less frequently in the sigmoid, tending to decrease in frequency as the proximal colon is reached. They vary in size and shape and may be sessile or pedunculated. They are most common in young and middle-aged adults. They are more prevalent in severe and destructive chronic cases and they are also encountered in the early fulminating cases. Most pseudopolyps are discrete or occur in clusters. Sometimes large areas of the colon may be studded with pseudopolyps with low, rounded surfaces, giving the mucosa a cobblestone appearance. The changes exhibit a mottled, honeycomb and mosaic pattern because of the numerous small rounded formations, projecting into the lumen. This condition is called pseudopolyposis.

Haustral abnormalities are classical but not specific. In the earliest stages no haustral abnormalities may be observed.

An increased haustration presents a smoothly undulating contour. It may resemble the edge of a sheet of corrugated iron. It is associated with irregular thickening of the haustra. As early as 1924 Kantor emphasized the "row of sausages" appearance seen in postevacuation films or in the film of the colon obtained six hours after ingestion of barium. He postulated that this was a sign of chronic nonspecific inflammation or irritation. According to Williams these corrugations are probably due to normal muscular contractions.

Poor muscular haustra may also be present and, according to Dick and co-workers (1959), they are associated with some colonic narrowing with submucosal inflammation and fibrosis.

An evaluation of the presacral space and of the prominent transverse valves in the rectum is significant for the degree of severity of the inflammatory process in the rectum. The rectosacral distance is usually 0.5 cm and any value above 0.7 in children and 1 cm in adults must be considered pathologic. Any inflammatory disease of the pelvis may produce widening of the space, as may infiltration of the tumors.

The rectal valves – Houston's valves – are usually three semilunar transverse folds, composed of mucosa and circular muscle fibers. They vary in number, size and location. At least one – Kohlrausch's fold, assumed to be the middle one – is seen constantly projecting from the right anterior aspect of the rectum and located at the level of the bladder. In the presence of inflammatory processes in the rectum, they may be destroyed or altered, varying from slight thickening and blunting to complete obliteration. These changes are not reversible, and, once established, the folds never again become entirely normal roentgenologically. The valves of Houston are of a dull hue and are depressed, their rounded edges having lost their sharp contour. Close scrutiny of the mucous membrane will reveal minute discrete capillary hemorrhages upon the generalized inflammatory process.

A correlation between the degree of increase in the rectosacral soft-tissue space, the destruction or alteration of the transverse valves and the course of the ulcerative colitis showed that the extent of the inflammatory changes in the wall and the severity of the disease are generally parallel. Preoperative knowledge of these changes is very important to the surgeon.

At first the whole colon is usually uniformly of smaller caliber than normal but can be distended in a normal way by increase in intraluminar pressure. Later the narrowing of the colon is constant and then there is severe submucosal fibrosis. The contractility is usually reduced in those colons showing narrowing and fibrosis but good contraction is occasionally seen even in the presence of marked narrowing and severe fibrosis.

In advanced cases the colon presents a true narrowing and a fixed configuration, indicating stiffness. The outlines are smooth, there are no haustrations; there is considerable shortening, resulting in downward displacement and uncoiling of the flexures resulting in a characteristic "lead pipe colon". The mucosa may be atrophic, degenerated or may have disappeared completely. The wall is thick and fibrosed and feels stiff and indurated. The pipestem colon is evident, but varying degrees of stiffness may be asymmetrical and may appear in one segment of the colon only.

Stiffness is associated not only with a short contracted colon but may also be present in an apparently dilated and redundant one. All of these changes are due to varying degrees of submucosal edema and fibrosis.

Roentgen Diagnosis

Every patient suspected of having ulcerative colitis should have an x-ray examination. It is especially important today, when there is such an increased interest in the diagnosis and treatment of ulcerative colitis. This is due to the introduction of new therapeutic methods and more active surgery. The clinicians are now inclined to refer their patients for operation at a relatively early stage. It is obvious that this tendency places increasing demands on diagnostic roentgenology. The clinician wants to have definite information of the nature of any change and preferably whether or not such a change is reversible. The roentgen study is also of value in the complications and sequelae of ulcerative colitis. Repeated examinations or regular follow-up will assist in determining the progress or regression of the disease: ulcerative colitis is dynamic, with exacerbations and remissions which may considerably alter the roentgenologic signs.

The old method using a conventional barium enema revealed several roentgenologic signs, each

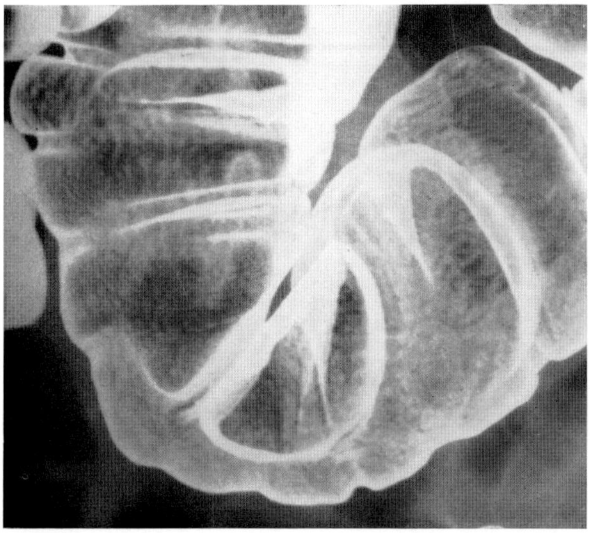

Fig. 77 a) ♂ 15 years. X-ray 21/4/72. Normal mucosal relief.

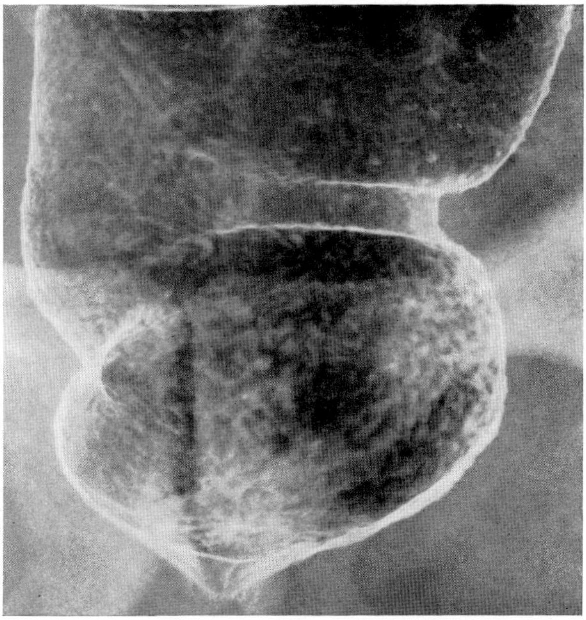

Fig. 77 b) ♂ 56 years. X-ray 8/8/55. A somewhat irregular, fine granular relief with increased distance between the contrast stripes. By sigmoidoscopy a mildly swollen red mucous membrane.

by itself not diagnostic, but suggestive as a group. The first roentgenologic indications of ulcerative colitis with that method are, according to Poppel and Beranbaum (1957), small smooth peaks, spikes or serrations, produced by barium between swollen mucosal folds. The projections are irregularly spaced and of different sizes but are usually not more than 1 to 3 mm in depth. The authors claimed that this change may be present in acute exudative colitis of any disease, including ulcerative colitis.

They alleged that these changes antedated ulcerations.

It was, however, often found that the conventional barium enema missed up to as many as 15 percent of cases with clear clinical and sigmoidoscopic evidence of colitis. By the use of the modification of the double contrast method this discrepancy has been eliminated.* This method can reveal even very early colitis. Even slight swelling, reddening and readily bleeding lesions can thus be recognized (Figs. 77a, b). Such small lesions show a somewhat irregular, finely granular surface and the distance between the normally 1 mm broad contrast stripes is somewhat increased. The picture is clearly abnormal. The mucosa appears nodular.

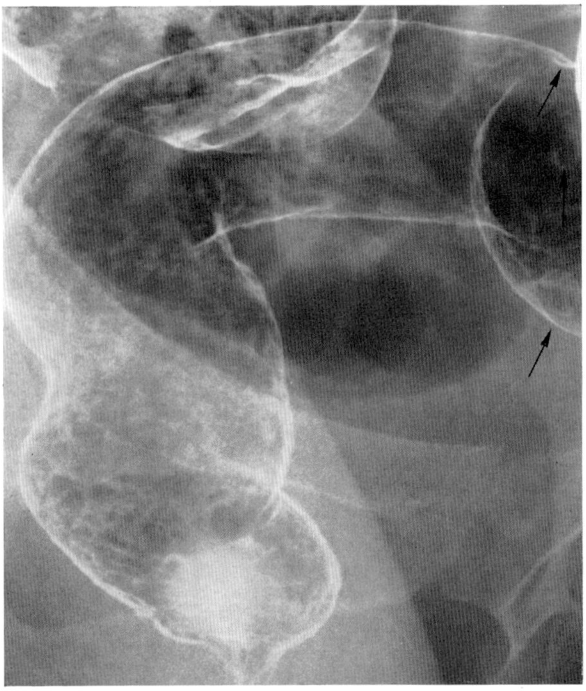

Fig. 78 a) ♀ 46 years. Ulcerative colitis. X-ray 14/5/62. Nodular mucosal pattern in rectum. Some small polyps at rectosigmoid junction.

* It should be observed that we do not use laxatives the day before or the actual day of the examination if we know the patient has ulcerative colitis, but we do give these patients atropine. The examination of patients with ulcerative colitis has never been attended by any complications, and the slight irritation sometimes occurring in association with the examination, is often followed by a period of several weeks, during which the symptoms are less severe than before the x-ray examination.

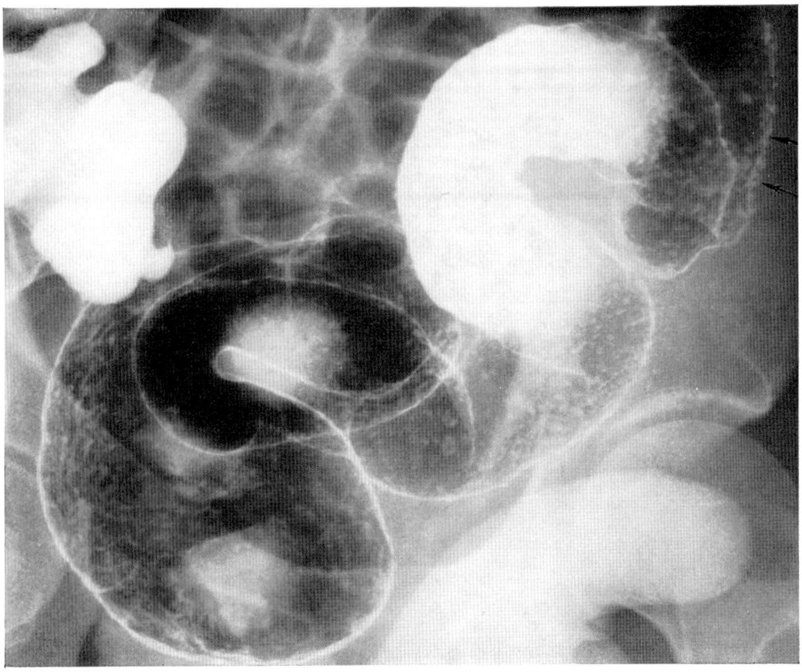

Fig. 78 b) ♂ 26 years. Ulcerative colitis. X-ray 14/12/70. More advanced irregular nodular pattern in rectum and sigmoid with small ulcerations in sigmoid.

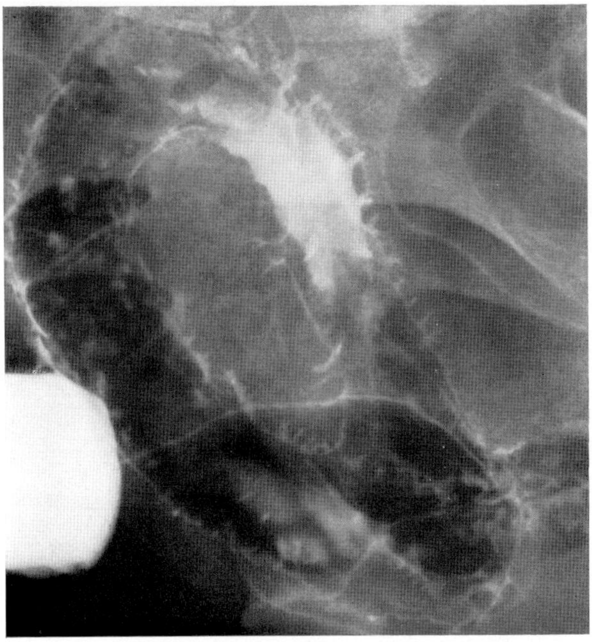

Fig. 78 c) ♀ 28 years. Ulcerative colitis. X-ray 15/10/70. Very narrowed sigmoid with multiple ulcerations, appearing as specks en face and as spikes in profile.

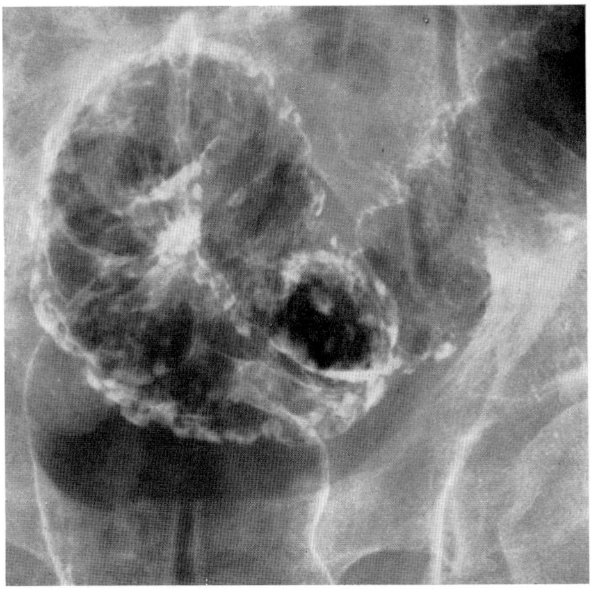

Fig. 78 d) ♂ 58 years. Ulcerative colitis. X-ray 15/10/70. In upper part of rectum and sigmoid nodular pattern with multiple deep ulcerations. Many with collar-stud configuration with tendency to coalesce. Double contour.

Simpkins and Stevenson (1972) in order to assess the accuracy of this modification in reflecting the sigmoidoscopic findings, examined 125 patients (60 with ulcerative colitis, eight with Crohn's disease and 57 with normal sigmoidoscopic

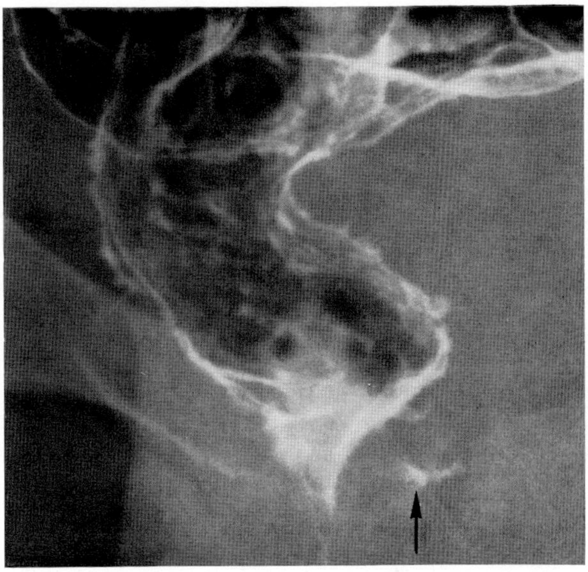

Fig. 78 e) ♀ 25 years. Ulcerative colitis. X-ray 24/9/63. Significantly narrowed and shortened rectum with coarsely nodular pattern and small ulcerations.

findings) using this method. They found that the state of the rectal mucosa was roentgenographically assessed correctly in 121 of 125 patients, an overall error of 3.2 percent. These authors stressed that the method showed the extent of even very early lesions including those above sigmoidoscopic level and thus verified the findings in the Malmö material. This is important because, according to de Dombal (1968), it is the extent of the affection that determines the late prognosis.

He also claimed that the rectal mucosal changes are both more sensitive and more reliable than absence of Houston's valves, which was noted in 43 percent, an increased recto sacral distance, which was noted in 3 percent, and a decreased rectal caliber, which was seen in 23 percent. These changes are not specific of ulcerative colitis. They may also occur in other inflammatory conditions.

If ulcerative colitis progresses, the inflammatory changes of the mucosa increase in severity. The distance between the contrast stripes increases and the irregularities are more striking. The mucosal pattern becomes nodular. Sometimes the picture leaves the impression of small polyps (Fig. 78a).

Further progress is characterized by the appearance of small ulcerations. They are first seen as punctate projections from the intestinal wall or

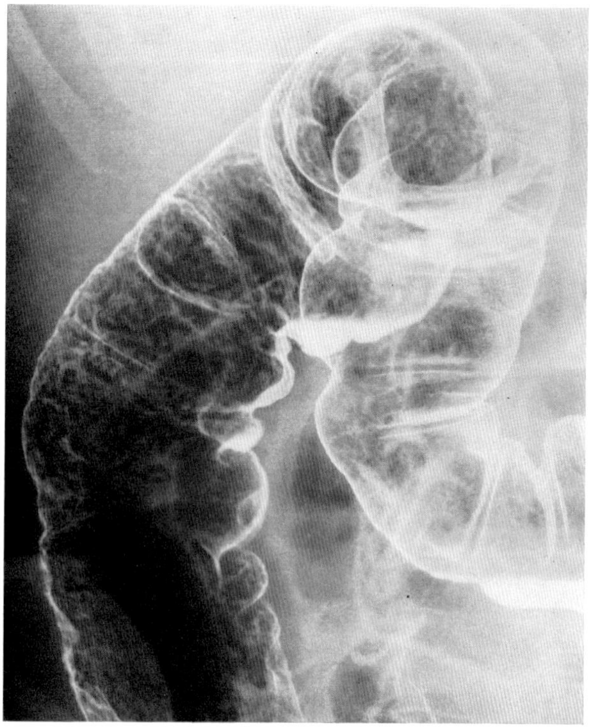

Fig. 79 ♂ 60 years. Ulcerative colitis. X-ray 2/12/69. In ascending colon a relatively fine nodular pattern without haustration. In transverse colon normal mucosal pattern and normal haustration.

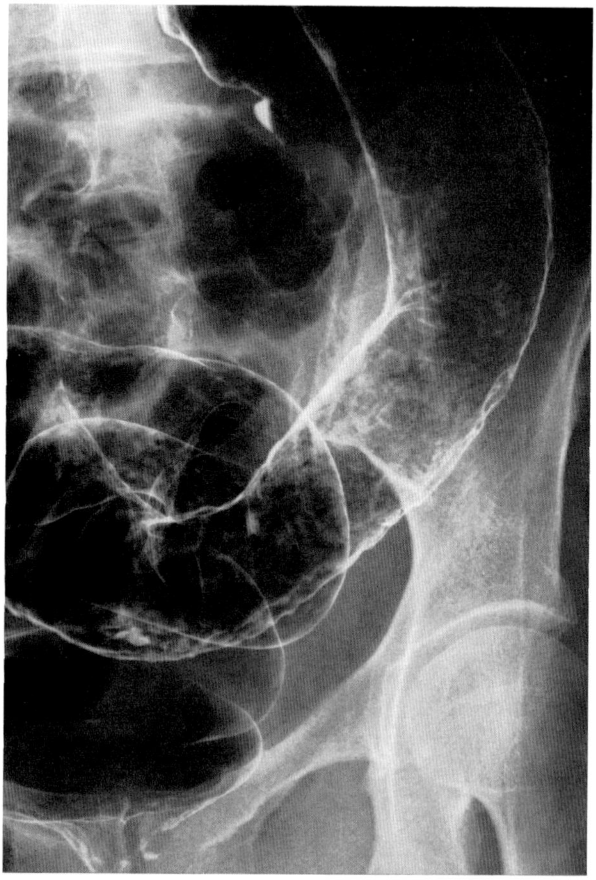

Fig. 80 ♀ 47 years. Ulcerative colitis. X-ray 3/8/70. Nodular mucosal pattern. No ulcerations, but a double contour along the lateral wall.

as small specks, depending on their orientation relative to the x-ray beam (Fig. 78b).

If they advance still further, the ulcerations become deeper and the mucosal changes coarser; the intestinal lumen often becomes narrower (Fig. 78c).

The ulcerations sometimes assume a collar stud appearance with their flattened bases along the external intestinal wall. They often tend to coalesce, then giving rise to a continuous track of barium along the bowel contour and connected with the lumen at several points. This track varies in length from a few to 30 centimeters (Fig. 78d).

In more advanced cases the rectum is narrowed and shortened. The mucosal relief is sparse and often completely atrophic. But in the event of exacerbations the pattern is often nodular and sometimes also shows small ulcerations (Fig. 78e).

Ulcerative colitis usually starts in the rectum and spreads upwards. Sometimes it involves the entire colon. In double contrast roentgenograms it is possible to follow this spread above sigmoidoscopic level. The mucosal changes and ulcerations are well defined as in the rectum. Sometimes the spread is limited to certain areas. In Fig. 79, for example, it is confined to the ascending colon; in Fig. 80, to the sigmoid and the distal part of the descending colon; and in Fig. 81, the entire colon is involved. In the last case the mucosal changes are less striking in the rectum than in the rest of the intestine.

The nodular pattern may become more or less coarse and vary from one part of the intestine to another. In advanced cases the nodules are crowded and separated only by very narrow stripes of contrast medium. The nodules often vary somewhat in size and then the condition is referred to as pseudopolyposis (Fig. 82). It has formerly been claimed that the pattern of pseudopolyposis can be distinguished from that of the cobblestone pattern of Crohns' disease because the pseudopolyps are rounder.

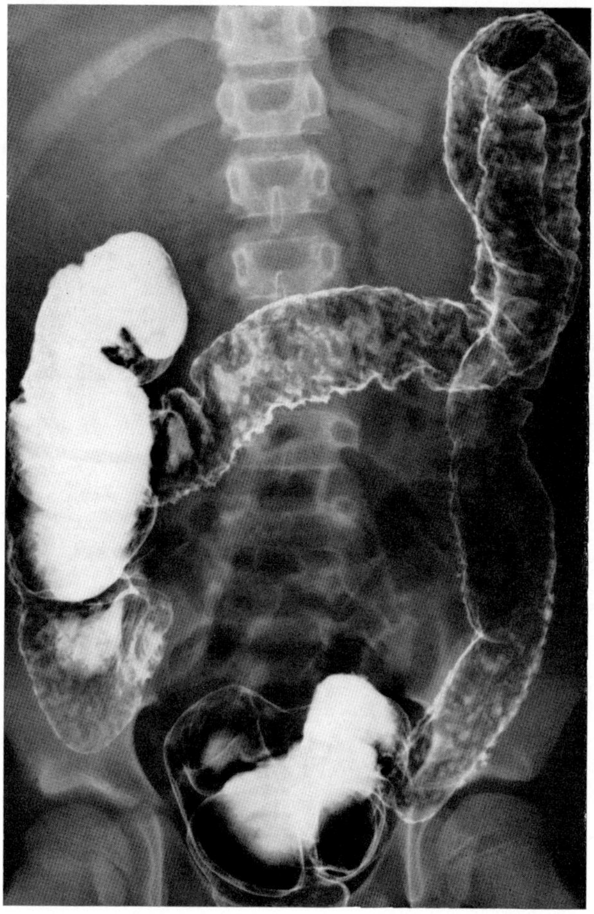

Fig. 81 ♂ 12 years. Ulcerative colitis. X-ray 12/2/59. Irregular nodular pattern with small ulcerations in the whole colon.

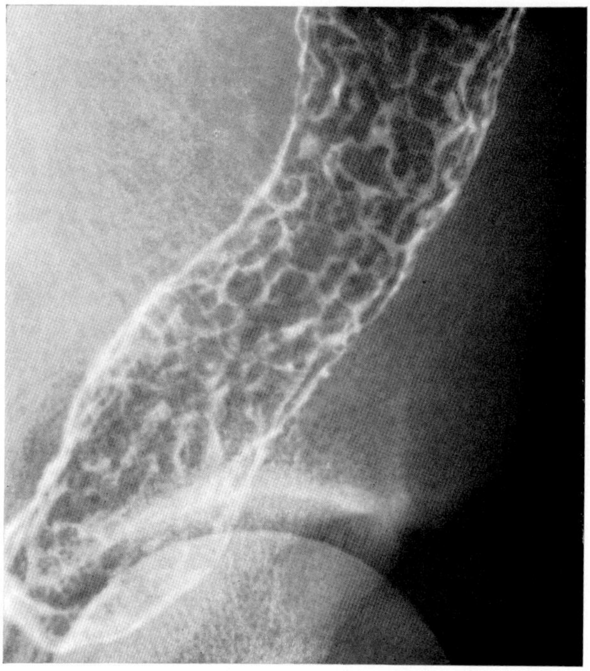

Fig. 82 ♂ 14 years. Ulcerative colitis. X-ray 12/8/71. Pseudopolyposis.

However, we have not found that this difference alone permits a firm differential diagnosis. However, in Crohn's disease the roentgenogram shows fine typical transverse stripes along the edges of the cobblestone pattern and these stripes can decide the diagnosis.

In advanced cases, pronounced narrowing, shortening and rigidity of the colon may develop and give the colon the appearance of a lead-pipe (Fig. 83b). The configuration of a lead-pipe colon is fixed; there is no uncoiling of the flexures, there are no haustra and the mucosal pattern is one of atrophy. Even this stage may develop fairly quickly (Figs. 83a and b).

This possibility of following the appearance and spread of the mucosal changes in detail means that we now have a refined diagnostic method.

Complications

Acute and chronic ulcerative colitis are prone to be attended by serious complications and the prognosis varies largely with the extent to which the complications can be prevented or controlled.

Acute Toxic Megacolon

Acute toxic dilatation of the colon offers serious problems. The pathogenesis of toxic segmental dilatation is unknown. It may be produced by severe disruption of the muscular coats of the bowel, by a disturbance of the symmetric plexus or perhaps by hypokalemia, which is very common. It may also follow treatment with glucocorticoids and ACTH. It is produced by accumulation of gas and discharges in the colon and in the small bowel. It may occur at any time during acute or chronic ulcerative colitis. This abdominal distension is a most alarming feature, and has been reported to occur in 2–8 percent of all cases in some series. The distended and tender abdomen suggests actual or imminent perforation. This complication has been reported as fatal with a frequency of 18 to 35 percent.

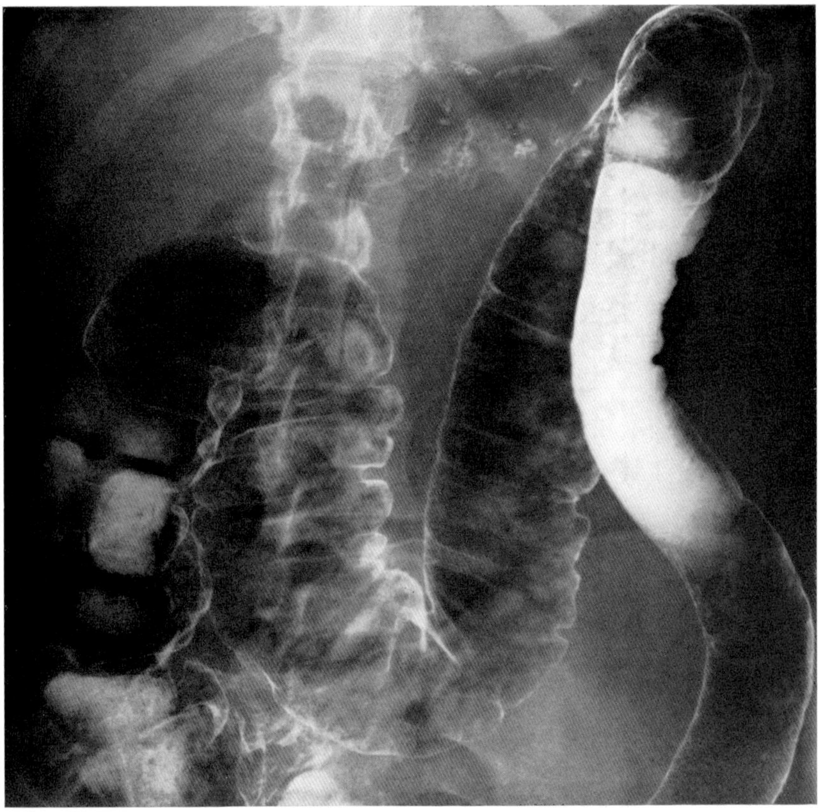

Fig. 83 ♂ 29 years:
a) X-ray 20/2/56. Normal appearance.

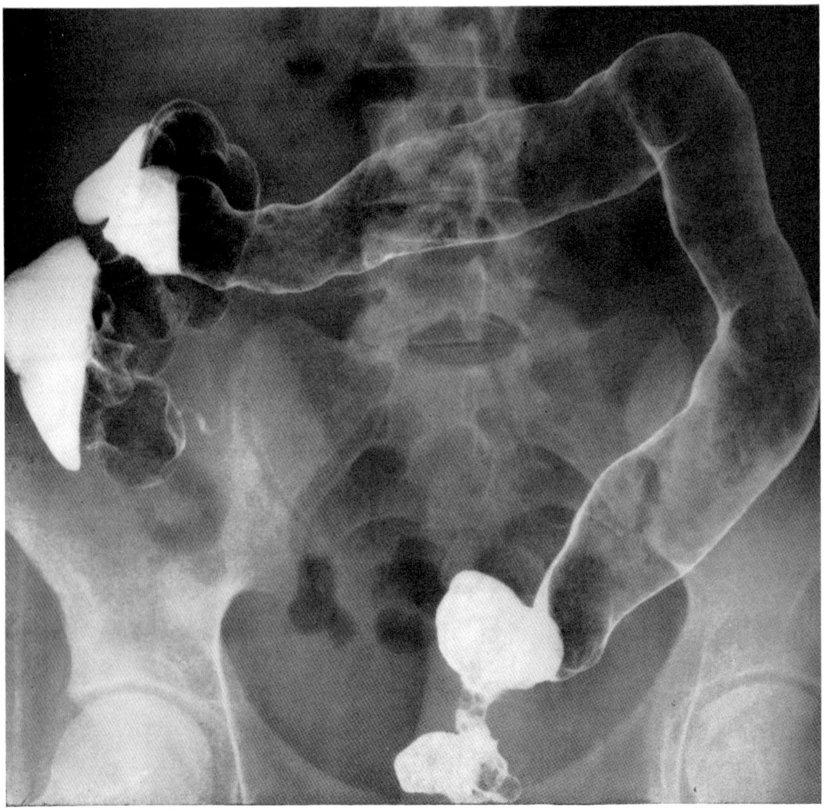

Fig. 83 b) X-ray 21/11/59. Same patient. Now lead-pipe colon.

The distension is most marked in the transverse colon; it is seldom seen in the rectum. It can be diagnosed by examination of a plain x-ray film of the abdomen. It may be an extremely large colon, measuring more than 10 cm across. There are few, but long, fluid levels. No remarkable redundancy or overlapping of the large bowel's gas shadow is seen because the dilated transverse colon is not elongated. Thickened inflamed mucosa may form irregular nodules, which protrude into the air-filled lumen and render the outline of the gas shadow irregular, nodular or scalloped. The nodular line may be seen not only along the margin of the bowel, but may be a striking feature in the thickening of the semilunar folds, provided they have not been affected by preexisting chronic colitis.

Haustral sacculations may be entirely absent. A barium enema is unnecessary. Occasionally such an examination is done but should preferably be avoided owing to the fragility of the colon.

Abscess and Fistulae

Ulcerative colitis is sometimes complicated by pericolic and perirectal abscesses, but inflammatory fistulae are rarely seen. Anal crypts may be infected and cause serious and painful perianal fistulae. Such a fistula should be treated gingerly. Fistulae above the rectum, resulting from slow perforation locally into neighboring viscera (the ileum, the stomach and other viscera) usually require surgical treatment.

Strictures

Strictures in ulcerative colitis is uncommon. According to Marshak (1963), they occur in only 1 percent of all cases. Dombal and others (1968), however, have identified strictures in 11.2 percent, mostly in the long-standing cases.

The most common site of the stricture is the rectum, where it usually assumes an annular or short tubular form, but any portion of the large bowel may be the site of narrowing. The left colon (Fig. 84) is affected more often than the right, but, according to Marshak, the ileocecal valve is also a common site of involvement. Long stretches of narrowing, sometimes 2 feet or more, are common. Segmental areas of narrowing are less frequent.

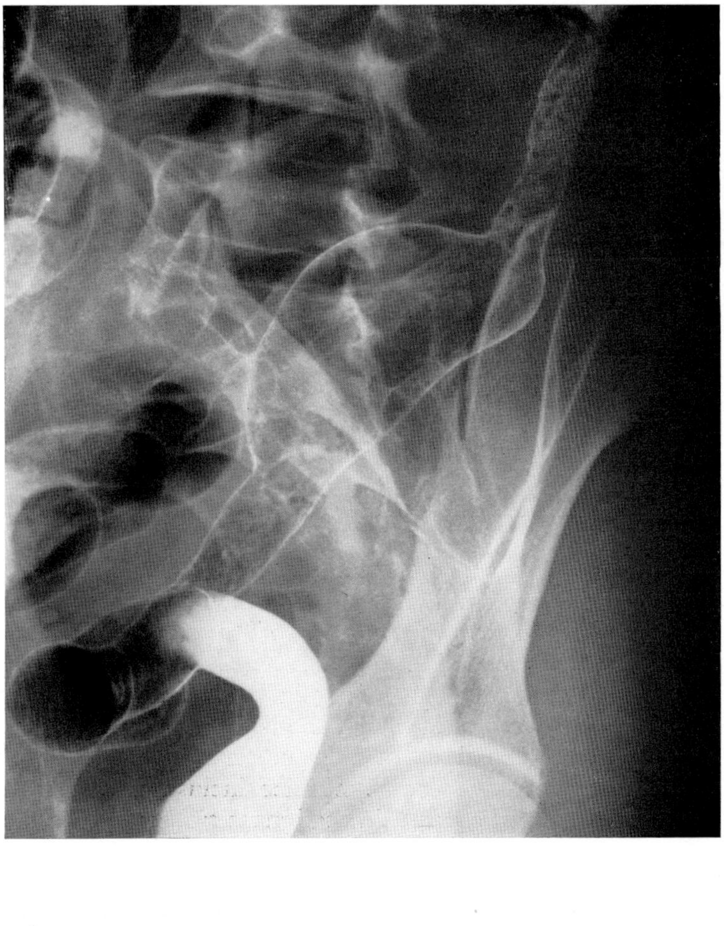

Fig. 84 ♂ 37 years. Ulcerative colitis. X-ray 9/5/67. Stenosis of descending colon in patient with ulcerative colitis. Pathologico-anatomically no signs of malignant disease.

Strictures are due to an organic stiff narrowing of the lumen, which may cause partial obstruction or scar tissue practically obliterating the lumen of the bowel. They are the result of the healing process with its formation of fibrous tissue. The lumen in the area of stricture is irregular and eccentric.

Benign inflammatory stricture of the colon is uncommon in patients with ulcerative colitis. Strictures developing in the colon of these patients must be regarded as signs of carcinoma, until the contrary is proved.

Perforarion

Perforation into the free peritoneal cavity is an uncommon complication; it is sometimes seen in acute dilatation of the colon in the fulminating stages owing to thinning of the ulcerated wall of the colon. A more common complication is perforation with abscess formation or development of a fistula between loops of colon or between colon and the small bowel, vagina or bladder. According to Simon et al. (1962), a characteristic roentgen sign of preperforative acute dilatation of the colon is the presence of a zone of translucency, outlining the serosal border of the distended colon. The authors believe that these radiolucent stripes reflect a submucosal accumulation of gas secondary to intramural fistulization resulting from increased permeability of the diseased mucosa. Such extraluminal gas may be seen as irregular stripes – two to four mm thick – of radiolucency of the bowel wall. These collections of gas must be distinguished from the presumably normal pericolic fat stripes, which are usually thinner, longer, more regular and continuous.

Ulcerative Colitis and Cancer

Bargen (1930) was first to demonstrate a relationship between carcinoma and ulcerative colitis. Evidence of the relationship of the two diseases was published in a report of the American Cancer Society in 1959, wherein it is stated that there are large inclusion bodies in the cytoplasm of mucosal cells of the colon of patients with ulcerative colitis. Similar inclusion bodies have been observed in malignant polyps of the colon. Further evidence of the tendency of the disease to become complicated by malignancy is the fact that in ulcerative colitis, only too frequently, carcinoma develops after the disease has been in progress for 10 years or more and patients are usually not more than 35 years of age when the cancer becomes manifest.

Incidence

Opinions concerning the incidence of cancer associated with chronic ulcerative colitis differ widely. Felsen and Wolarsky (1949) wrote that the alleged association of the two diseases was a myth. In their series of 855 patients not a single case of carcinoma had occurred, and Snapper in 1949 corroborated their opinion. But nowadays the incidence has been shown to be considerably higher than in the general population (0.06 percent). Bargen, for example, estimated that the calculated risk of cancer of the colon developing into ulcerative colitis was 30 times more common than in corresponding age groups in the general population, and Brooke (1961) alleged that ulcerative colitis was a precancerous condition.

The duration of the disease is of paramount importance. Colcock (1954), for example, found an incidence as high as 30 percent in patients who had had the disease for 10 years or more; Garlock (1959), 36 percent if they had had the disease 12 years or longer; and Counsell and Dukes (1952) 45 percent. In Edling's (1959) series the average duration, until the discovery of malignant degeneration was 15.4 years, in Goldgraber's series (1965), 11.2 years and in Fennessy's series (1966) 16.9. These figures are remarkably similar to the duration of colitis reported from other institutions in the U.S.A. and elsewhere.

If the onset of colitis is early in life, i.e. in childhood or adolescence, cancer occurs sooner and with greater frequency.

It has also been alleged that carcinoma is particularly liable to arise in the colon with extensive involvement and is less likely to occur or does not occur more frequently than in the intact colon, when the changes are limited to the distal segment of the colon.

The mean age at the time of detection of carcinoma in Fennessy's series (1968) was 37.7 years, in striking contrast with those individuals with an intact colon, who develop carcinoma at an average age of 57.8 years.

Distribution

Some authors are of the opinion that the distribution of these carcinomas was similar to that which is generally accepted; that those lesions are most common in the rectum, rectosigmoid and sigmoid flexure. Goldgraber (1959), however, found a more even distribution over the colon, and Edling (1961) found only 15 percent of the growths to be situated at the rectosigmoid junction and 85 percent elsewhere in the colon. Edling's study indicated thus that the malignant tumors are distributed in a manner opposite to large bowel tumors in general.
The multiplicity of the tumors in these patients is also noteworthy. Two or more primary carcinomas arise in 34 percent (Fennessy 1968); Bargen, Bargen and Dockerty (1958) detected multiple tumors in 4.6 percent of a large series of patients with an intact colon.

Clinical Symptoms

According to Brooke (1961), there are only two symptoms which point to cancerous change – pain and obstruction. Both are symptoms of a growth which has advanced beyond the possibility of cure by surgery. Other authors claim that the occurrence of new symptoms – progressive loss of weight, weakness, heavy bleeding and lumps palpated by the patient – point in the same direction. Most patients experienced moderately severe symptoms of colitis (56 percent). The symptoms were severe in 33 percent and mild in the remainder.

Etiology

Edling and many others are convinced of a definite relationship between malignant degeneration and ulcerative colitis. They base their opinion on the high incidence of cancer, its development at much earlier ages and the difference in distribution from bowel tumors in general.
Although it is difficult to explain the sequence of events in a patient with ulcerative colitis later complicated by carcinoma, it is apparent that continued regeneration of epithelium and the presence of abundant new vascular tissue are important factors. Dukes (1958) has called attention to the attempt on the part of the cells of the epithelial lining to grow into and re-epithelialize an evacuated abscess cavity. Occasionally, during this process, nests of cells or glandular epithelium may become trapped and buried in the submucosa. Repair occurs above, sealing off these young cells. According to Dukes, this "seed and soil" relationship could well be a predisposing factor in the development of carcinoma in chronic ulcerative colitis.
In this connection pseudopolyps have attracted much attention, particularly as carcinoma has been found in 16.3 percent of patients with pseudopolypoid changes. The concept of the precancerous nature of pseudoadenomatous polyps was advanced as early as 1927 by Yeomans. Swartz (1949) accepted this concept and emphasized that there must be either a direct relationship between pseudopolyps or the predisposition of pseudopolyps to carcinoma. Dawson (1921) and Castleman (1962) felt that pseudopolyps can become malignant either directly or after transformation into adenomas or villous papillomas, even if it is probable that it is a rare event.
But most authors do not believe that the development of cancer is related to the presence of inflammatory pseudopolyps. Gelber (1955) reasons that when the structure of the pseudopolyp is compared with that of the adenomatous polyp, one can only assume that it could not undergo the same morphological changes. The marked proliferative activity of the cells of an adenomatous polyp compared with that of the pseudopolyp (with its marked inflammatory infiltration and edema in the mucosa) represents an entirely different type of cellular activity. Hardy and Bulmer (1933) are also of the opinion that pseudopolyps carry little risk of potential malignancy and Swinton and Warren (1927) refuse to accept the possibility that the pseudopolyps are precancerous. Otani and Snapper (1952) believe that a malignant neoplasm is coexistent and not secondary to the inflammatory polyps and that an adenomatous polyp is the probable site of origin. Ganshorn (1935), like us in Malmö, has noted a high incidence of polyps in ulcerative colitis and has shown that carcinomatous changes are more common in patients with adenomatous hyperplasia of the mucous membrane.

Pathology

Some authors distinguish three types of these tumors. Firstly a very malignant carcinoma, which develops from widely separated foci, spreads rapidly and literally ensheathes the colon, so that the entire colonic wall becomes a thick infiltrated tube. Secondly, a type which originates from isolated and local foci of epithelial cells. Although the colon may be the site of several primary neoplasms, surgical cure is possible if the condition is diagnosed resonably early. Thirdly, a form in which early neoplastic changes may occur in the mucosal tags of a diseased rectum; similar lesions may be discovered during routine histopathologic examination of surgical specimens after colectomy. These tumors are invariably of a low grade of malignancy, and surgical removal or electrocoagulation will result in complete eradication.

In a bowel with severe, destructive ulcerative colitis, it is apparent that continued regeneration of epithelium exceeds the normal requirements. The second important factor in the development of carcinoma concerns its relationship to tissue repair. What actually happens to the normal process of tissue repair in patients with chronic ulcerative colitis who develop carcinoma is not properly understood. It seems probable that repair proceeds without control.

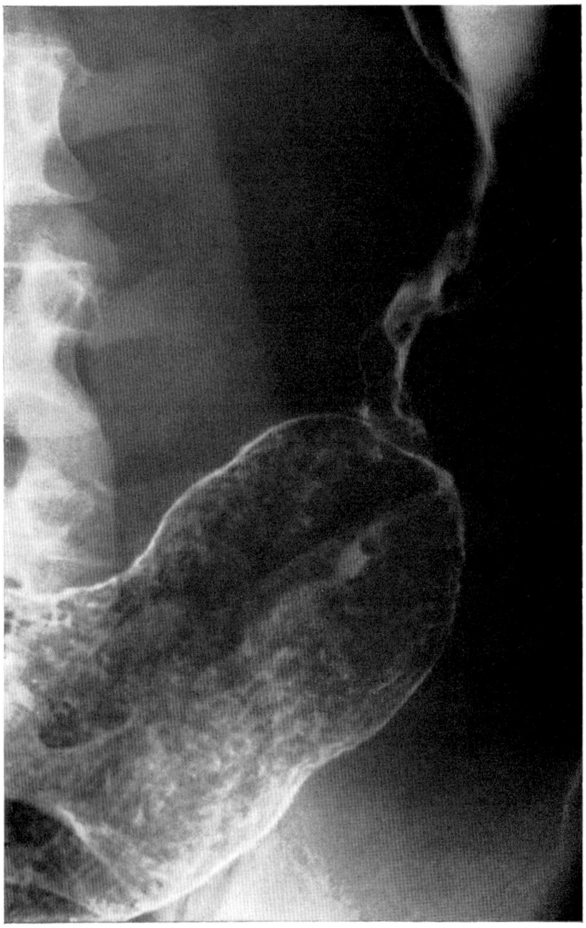

Fig. 85 ♂ 28 years. Ulcerative colitis. X-ray 24/3/58. Annular cuff-like carcinoma in descending colon. Nodular pattern distally – ulcerative colitis.

Macroscopically, the lesion may be constricting, annular, sessile, polypoid or scirrhous. The constricting carcinoma most frequently encountered is characteristically long. The lumen of the bowel is narrowed, and its ragged and irregular lumen shows numerous small, polyp-like projections. The ends of the constricted segments are cone-shaped. The constriction may be concentric or eccentric, but it is always irregular. There is usually no sharp border between carcinoma and contiguous mucosa.

In scirrhous carcinoma there may be no clinical or roentgen signs of neoplasm. Because of replacement of the mucosa by layers of cancer cells, the bowel has a relatively flat surface, which is roentgenologically indistinguishable from the denuded mucosa of burned-out chronic ulcerative colitis. When some segmental narrowing is present, differentiation between carcinoma and stricture is difficult, since the flat surface of the lumen of the narrowed segment of the bowel may look exactly the same in scirrhous carcinoma and stricture.

Roentgen Diagnosis

The roentgen diagnosis of these carcinomas is sometimes difficult. The roentgenologic appearance of the colon with ulcerative colitis has no characteristic permitting prediction or exclusion of the subsequent development of cancer. The most common form is the long constricting lesions with coneshaped ends. Fig. 85 shows such a case with a granular mucosa and, in the middle of the descending colon, a stenosis 4 cm long. The distinct border of this cuff-like stenosis and the ragged and rigid mucosa suggests a malignant neoplasm rather than stenosis due to inflammation. If the stenosis is due to inflammation, the outline is usually smoother and the mucosa has a different pattern. According to some investigators, it is not possible to differentiate between a neoplasm and an inflammatory lesion preoperatively, but the results of roentgen examination have improved since the introduction of the new modification of the double contrast method except regarding the scirrhous variety, in which the lesions may often resemble strictures.

Prognosis

The earlier the onset of ulcerative colitis in life, the more severe the attacks, the poorer the control, and the more likely cancer is to develop. The frequency of death from malignant neoplasm is highest among the patients with the earliest onset of chronic ulcerative colitis and decreases sharply with increasing age. More than 50 percent of those who later develop carcinoma have symptoms of ulcerative colitis before the age of 40. The carcinoma develops relatively early in life and the grade of malignancy according to Broder's method is generally higher than in patients with carcinoma who do not have ulcerative colitis.

Differential Diagnosis

Familial Polyposis

The roentgen findings may be similar to those in pseudopolyposis, but inflammatory changes, absent haustrations, shortening, narrowing and tubular configuration and ulcerations are not present in familial polyposis.

Chronic Radiation Effect

Strictures following radiation treatment of carcinoma of the cervix or the body of the uterus may not begin until several months to many years later. The most common site of stricture is the rectosigmoid and sigmoid. The segment is usually longer than might be expected with a carcinoma and its ends taper. Mucosal ulcerations are common. They usually circumscribe the diseased area. Mucosal and submucosal edema may produce "saw-tooth" and thumbprint effects along the body of the stricture. Knowledge of early radiation treatment and of the site and the features of the lesion help to differentiate it from primary tumors or metastases.

Endometriosis

In endometriosis bowel involvement is more common than generally believed. It is most common in the rectum and sigmoid and should be considered in women who have rectal pain or tenesmus associated with menstruation. Only rarely does rectal bleeding occur during menstruation.

Roentgenologically the lesions are usually covered by mucosa; they are smooth and sometimes multiple. The changes may be mistaken, both clinically and roentgenologically, for benign or malignant tumors.

Ulcerative Colitis in Children

The modification of the double contrast method is also useful in the diagnosis of ulcerative colitis in children. The method is both effective and reliable. As the clinical picture in a child is much more serious than the proctoscopic finding, adequate roentgen examination is of great value, particularly for deciding whether an operation is indicated and if so, the choice of surgical treatment and the extent of the operation.

In the early stage, the initial examination often reveals small shallow ulcers scattered over the areas of the mucosa of the colon. However, in several of the very early cases in our material no ulcers were seen. Instead the mucosa was covered with minute, granular lesions, only visible on the contrast-coated bowel surface, viewed en face. On close inspection very small somewhat irregular rings were observed. Often the haustral markings and the folds of Kohlrausch were preserved. Later examinations usually revealed shallow, crowded ulcers. In the double contrast films they were visible not only as minute spiculae projecting into the bowel wall, but also as an irregular pattern on its mucosal surface. In some cases the ulcers deepened as the symptoms progressed, but in others they remained superficial for many months or even years. We have not seen them extend as deeply in children as they do in adults.

If the lesions progress, the haustra disappear as do the Kohlrausch's folds in the rectum. The intestine becomes shorter and assumes the well-known tube-like appearance without changes in caliber.

Several authors, such as Alford and associates (1963), claim that the roentgen changes usually begin in the rectum and extend upwards. In the Malmö material, however, the site and the extent of the disease in children differed widely from what is seen in adults. In as many as 95 percent the entire colon was involved already at the first roentgen examination, though the patients had had symptoms for at most a couple of weeks. Similar figures have been reported by Bargens and Kennedy (1941) 78 percent and by Lagercrantz (1955) 69 percent.

In almost all patients under 15 years, the lesions were equally severe in all the involved segments of the colon and even during periods of progress or regression the affected areas had a similar appearance throughout their length. Only in advanced cases, where strictures and mucosal destruction had developed, did the lesions differ from one segment to another.

In older patients (15 to 20 years of age) the lesions were generally much more marked in the rectum and the left half of the colon and faded as they extended cephalad. When the symptoms in this group regressed, healing usually began in the proximal segments. The last lesions to disappear were those situated in the sigmoid flexure and rectum.

The prognosis of ulcerative colitis in children is known to be gloomier than that of ulcerative colitis appearing in adult age. In childhood the frequency of complications is higher, especially local complications – polyps, strictures, fistulae – but also manifestations in other organs – growth retardation with underdeveloped epiphyses of the bones, nephritis, pyelitis, endocarditis etc. There is also a risk of cancer, which, according to Edling and associates, occurs in as many as 33 percent of all patients who have had ulcerative colitis for more than 15 years. Goldberg (1968) alleges, however, that treatment with hydrocortisone oil retention enemas has altered the prognosis. In the Malmö material also, the roentgen changes in relatively advanced cases sometimes regressed. The earlier opinion that the prognosis of the disease can be assessed from the findings made at the first roentgen examination does not hold for the disease in children.

11 Deformation of the Rectosigmoid Junction by External Endometriosis and Peritoneal Carcinomatosis

External endometriosis is a fairly common condition characterized by the extrauterine growth of endometrial tissue or possibly metaplastic tissue resembling endometrium. Circumscribed tumefaction may develop, but more often the process invades contiguous tissues with the formation of almost pathognomonically firm and rigid adhesions as well as a marked degree of puckering and scarring. Despite the infiltrative mode of growth, the mucosa of the rectum and sigmoid colon is seldom invaded. The pelvic peritoneum, the rectovaginal septum and sigmoid colon are clinically important sites of predilection. The tendency of the adhesions to undergo fibrosis and to contract is suspicious; even consequent folding and angulation of the bowel has been observed (Tagart 1959).

The roentgenographic appearance is dependent upon the size and shape of the lesion of the aberrant endometrium. Roentgenography (Fig. 86) sometimes shows a peculiar deformity of the rectosigmoid junction. As a rule, it is demonstrable only in the lateral view (Wehlin and Theander 1961). It affects the anterior wall of the bowel below the sacral promontory. It appears as a blunt transverse ridge, about two to four cm in breadth, which projects backwards into the lumen and thus seems to exaggerate the normal curve of that part of the wall. The ridge is rounded and more or less well outlined, but as a rule its surface is not quite smooth. The ridge is resistant and usually prevents the passage of a sigmoidoscope. It sometimes resembles a polypoid tumor.

The deformity is fairly characteristic in women with pelvic endometriosis but not pathognomonic. Several kinds of pathologic processes outside the rectum may also deform this organ at various levels by causing a ridge-shaped protrusion of part of its wall into the lumen. The condition is usually called shelf-tumor irrespective of its actual nature.

Observations made during and after surgery have shown that the deformity in patients with pelvic endometriosis is due to contraction of the fibrous tissue at the rectosigmoid junction and is thus responsible for the occurrence and site of the deformity.

The same deformity can be seen also in peritoneal carcinomatosis (Theander, Wehlin and Langeland 1963). Since autopsy of such cases has failed to demonstrate any intramural growth of malignant tissue or of pressure exerted by some neighboring tumor or tumors and as more or

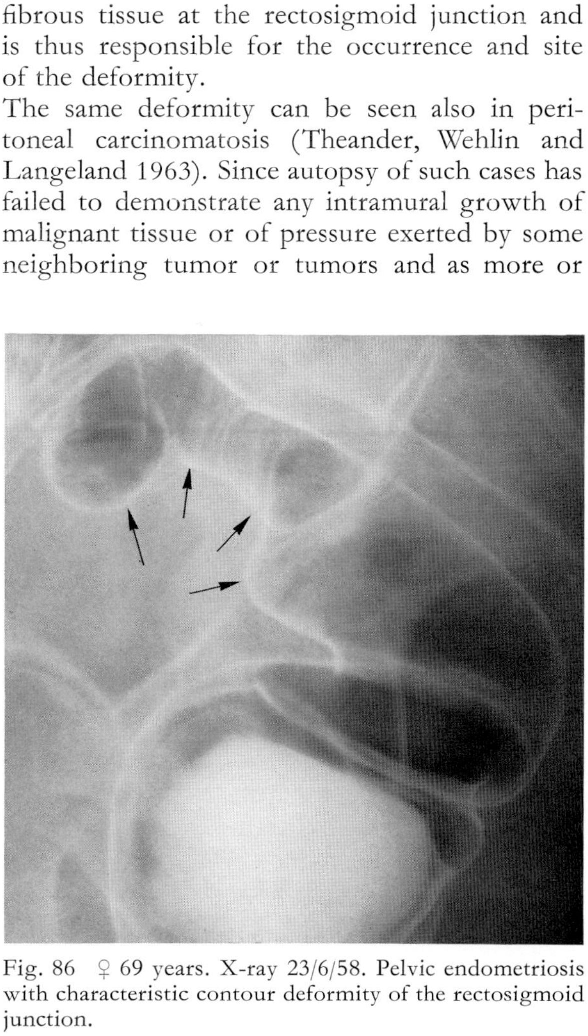

Fig. 86 ♀ 69 years. X-ray 23/6/58. Pelvic endometriosis with characteristic contour deformity of the rectosigmoid junction.

less marked fibrosis is known to be a constant feature of the resultant serosal lesion, it appears that in these cases too the junction deformity is related to the serosal fibrosis.

Other forms of pathologic processes outside the rectum, causing contracting adhesions in the pelvic, e.g. fibrosis following infections and radiotherapy, may also deform this organ at various levels by causing a ridge-shaped protrusion of its wall into the lumen.

It is important to distinguish this deformity from infiltration caused by primary carcinoma of the bowel, but despite the smooth outline and site of the change this is not always possible.

References

Ackerman, L. V.: Surgical pathology. Mosby, St. Louis 1953

Ackerman, L.V., J.A. Del Regato: Cancer. 3rd Edn. Mosby, St. Louis 1962

Alford, J.E., M.I. Rubin, J.K. McGregor: Chronic ulcerative colitis in children. Dis. Colon Rect. 6: 264–268, 1963

Almén, T.: Simple device for technical improvement of bowel examination of patients with colostomy. Brit. J. Radiol. 38: 75–76, 1965

Almy, T.P.: Diverticular disease of the colon – the new look. Gastroenterology 49: 109–112, 1965

D'Alo, R.: Aspecific inflammatory tumors of the large intestine. Radiol. Med. (Torino) 41: 959–980, 1955

Anderson, L.: Acute diverticulitis of the coecum. Surgery 22: 479–488, 1947

Andreassen, J.C.: Mucosal polyps of the colon and rectum: classification and relation to carcinoma. A study based on 9 years material with follow-up examinations. Acta chir. scand., Suppl. 396: 123–169, 1969

Andrén, L.: Ein Fall von Traktionsdivertikel im Kolon. Fortschr. Röntgenstr. 83: 594–595, 1955

Andrén, L., S. Frieberg: The relation of intestinal bleeding to polyps of the colon and rectum. Acta chir. scand. 112: 47–50, 1956

Andrén, L., S. Frieberg: Spontaneous regression of polyps of the colon in children. Acta radiol (Stockh.) 46: 507–510, 1956

Andrén, L., S. Frieberg: Roentgendiagnosis of the rectum. Gastroenterology 31: 566–570, 1956

Andrén, L., S. Frieberg: Frequency of polyps of the rectum and colon, according to age, and relation to cancer. Gastroenterology 36: 631–632, 1959

Andrén, L., S. Welin: Über die Häufigkeit von Kolonpolypen bei ulzeröser Kolitis. Fortschr. Röntgenstr. 92: 567–568, 1960

Andrén. L., S. Frieberg, S. Welin: Roentgen diagnosis of small polyps in the colon and rectum. Acta radiol. (Stockh.) 43: 201–208, 1955

Anton, H.C., J.H. Palmer: Corrugation of the colon: Its significance in ulcerative colitis. Brit. J. Radiol. 35: 762–768, 1962

Anton, H.C., D.H. Sutherland: Unusual presentation of segmental colitis. Brit. J. Radiol. 36: 33–39, 1963

Appelman, H.D.: Isolated diverticulitis of the sigmoid colon. Dis. Colon Rect. 13: 39–41, 1970

Appleman, R.M., R.J. Jackman: Regional enteritis. Proctoscopic clues in diagnosis. Dis. Colon Rect. 5: 361–363, 1962

Apsimon, H.T.: The single phase double contrast enema; a technique suitable for the average department. Clin. Radiol. 21: 188–194, 1970

Arfwidsson, F., N.G. Knock, L. Lehman et al.: Pathogenesis of multiple diverticula of the sigmoid colon in diverticular disease. Acta chir. scand., Suppl. 342: 1–68, 1964

Atwater, J.S., J.A. Bargen: Pathogenesis of intestina polyps. Gastroenterology 4: 395–408, 1945

Atwell, J.D., H.L. Duthie, J.C. Goligher: The outcome of Crohn's disease. Brit. J. Surg. 52: 966–972, 1965

Aurin, F.B., J.S. Marietta: Villous polyposis of the large intestine: A case report and review of the literature. Dis. Colon Rect. 4: 189–194, 1961

Bacon, H.E.: Ulcerative colitis. Lippincott, Philadelphia 1958

Bacon. H.E., J. Pezzutti: Granulomatous ileocolitis. J. Amer. med. Ass. 198: 1330–1334, 1966

Bacon, H.E., J. Laurens, A.R. Peale: Histopathology of adenomatous polyps of the colon and rectum, with special emphasis on relationship between adenoma and carcinoma. Surgery 29: 663–677, 1951

Barboka, C.J.: Diverticulosis and diverticulitis. Gastroenterology 34: 278–285, 1958

Bargen, J.A.: Inception of polyps of intestine; their association with and relationship to malignant disease. Proc. Mayo Clin. 15: 105–107, 1940

Bargen, J.A.: The nature of the carcinoma associated with ulcerative colitis. Dis. Colon Rect. 5, 356–360, 1962

Bargen, J.A.: Chronic ulcerative colitis: diagnostic and therapeutic problems: A lifelong study. Amer. J. Roentgenol. 99: 5–17, 1967

Bargen, J.A., M.W. Comfort: Association of chronic ulcerative colitis and multiple polyps. Ann. intern. Med. 4: 122–133, 1930

Bargen, J.A., R.P. Gage: Carcinoma and ulcerative colitis: prognosis. Gastroenterology 39: 385–393, 1960

Bargen, J.A., C.D.L. Cormar, C.F. Dixon: Early carcinoma of colon; nature and adequate treatment of small carcinomas. Arch Surg. 43: 192–208, 1941

Bartone, N.F., R.V. Grieco: Acute diverticulitis of the terminal ileum. J. Amer. med. Ass. 202: 1103–1106, 1967

Bartone, N.F., R.V. Grieco, A. Vasilles: A review of roentgen signs in lesions affecting the cecum. Amer. J. Roentgenol. 84: 285–305, 1960

Becker, W.: Zur Anwendung des Röntgenschen Verfahrens in der Medizin. Dtsch. med. Wschr. 22: 202–203, 1896

Becker, R., A. Oppenheimer: Zur Diagnose der Diverticulitis des Dickdarms. Röntgenpraxis 3: 1099–1101, 1931

Beekman, C.: Some important factors in the preparation of a barium enema. J. belge Radiol. 52: 210–219, 1969

Beer, E.: Some pathological and clinical aspects of acquired (false) diverticula of the intestine. Amer. J. med. Sci. 128: 135–145, 1904

Bell, J.C.: General considerations in the roentgen examination of the colon. Radiology 55: 20–23, 1950

Bell, J.C., J.B. Douglas: Roentgen ray diagnosis of malignant and potentially malignant lesions of colon and rectum. Radiology 51: 297–304, 1948

Bellin, A., P. Benoit, J. Aussage: Complications of diverticula of the sigmoid colon. Ann. Radiol. 7: 816–838, 1964
Bellman, H., H. Graetz: Differential diagnosis between diverticulitis tumour and carcinoma of the sigmoid colon. Zbl. Chir. 94: 241–254, 1969
Benetatos, S.: Étude radiologique des récidives postopératoires du cancer du côlon au niveau de l-anastomose termino-terminale. J. Radiol. Électrol. 41: 779–790, 1960
Bennet, J. M., A. Sands: Acute diverticulitis of the ascending colon. Report of three cases. Dis. Colon Rect. 4: 195–198, 1967
Beranbaum, S. L.: Roentgenologic diagnosis of idiopathic, non-specific ulcerative colitis, with special reference to early manifestations. Dis. Colon Rect. 7: 135–146 1964
Beranbaum, S. L.: Granulomatous colitis (Crohn's disease of colon). Differentiation from idiopathic ulcerative colitis. N. Y. med. J. 67: 244–247, 1967
Beranbaum, S. L., S. M. Ring: Ulcerative colitis engrafted upon diverticulitis. An evolutionary case history. Amer. J. Roentgenol. 104: 551–556, 1968
Beranbaum, S. L., M. Yaghmai, E. R. Beranbaum: Ulcerative colitis in association with diverticular disease of the colon. Radiology 85: 880–886, 1965
Beranbaum, S. L., J. Zausner, B. Lane: Diverticular disease of the right colon. Amer. J. Roentgenol. 115: 334–348, 1972
Bercoviez, Z. T.: Ulcerative colitis in older age patients. Gastroenterology 39: 28–33, 1960
Berge, T., G. Ekelund, C. Mellner, B. Pihl, A. Wenkert: Carcinoma of the colon and rectum in a defined population. Acta chir. scand., Suppl. 438: 1–86, 1973
Bergstermann, H.: Erfahrungen mit dem neuen Kontrastmittel für Irrigoskopien "Unibaryt rectal". Fortschr. Röntgenstr. 78: 354–356, 1953
Berman, L. G., D. Burdick, E. R. Heitzman, J. T. Prior: A critical reappraisal of sigmoid peridiverticulitis. Surg. Gynec. Obstet. 127: 481–491, 1968
Biancalana, L.: Diverticulose e diverticulite del Colon. Minerva med. 53: 381–385, 1962
Bickham jr, C. E.: Fistulous tracts with intestinal communication secondary to abscess formation in diverticulitis. Amer. J. Roentgenol. 79: 854–861, 1958
Binkley, G. E., D. A. Sunderland, C. Miller, M. Stearns, M. R. Deddish: Carcinoma arising in adenomas of colon and rectum. J. Amer. med. Ass. 148: 1465–1469, 1952
Birkner, R.: Über die Divertikulitis des Dickdarms, ihre Behandlungsmöglichkeiten und den Wert der Strahlenbehandlung. Strahlentherapie 78: 231–244, 1948
Blatt, L. J.: Polyps of the colon and rectum: incidence and distribution. Dis. Colon Rect. 4: 277–282, 1961
Blum, H. F.: On the mechanism of cancer induction by ultraviolet radiation. J. nat. Cancer Inst. 23: 337–342, 1959
Blumer, G.: The rectal shelf: a neglected rectal sign of value in diagnosis of obscure malignant and inflammatory diease within the abdomen. Albany med. Ann. 30: 1961, 1909
Bockus, H. L. V. Tachdjian, L. K. Ferguson, Y. Mouhran, C. Chamberlain: Adenomatous polyps of colon and rectum: its relation to carcinoma. Gastroenterology 41: 225–232, 1961
Bockus, H. L., B. C. Morson, R. H. Marshak, J. A. Bargen, B. Broke, S. B. Marshall, B. B. Crohn: Panel discussion of regional enterocolitis. Dis. Colon Rect. 8: 1–10, 1965
Bockus, H. L., J. L. A. Roth, E. Buchman, M. Kalser, W. R. Staub, A. Finkelstein, A. Valdes-Dapena: Life history of nonspecific ulcerative colitis: Relationship of prognosis to anatomical and clinical varietis. Gastroenterologia 86: 549–581, 1956
Bodart, P., C. Dive, G. van Trappen: Radiologic differences between ileocecal tuberculosis and Crohn's disease. Amer. J. dig. Dis. 6: 604–621, 1961
Boehme, E. J., P. J. Hansson: Carcinoma of the colon and rectum: site of growth of 1457 lesions. Surg. Clin. N. Amer. 26: 551–552, 1946
Boles, R. S., Ph. J. Hodes: Endometriosis of the small and large intestine. Gastroenterology 34: 367–380, 1958
Boles, R. S., S. M. Jorden: The clinical significance of diverticulosis. Gastroenterology 35: 579–582, 1958
Botsford, T. W., R. M. Zollinger jr: Diverticulitis of the colon. Surg. Gynec. Obstet. 128: 1209–1214, 1969
Boyd, C. E.: Polyps of the colon. New Orleans med. surg. J. 104: 92–96, 1951
Brahme, F.: Granulomatous colitis. Roentgenologic appearance and course of the lesions. Amer. J. Roentgenol. 99: 35–44, 1967
Brahme, F.: Early ulcerative colitis in children and adolescens. Dis. Colon Rect. 10: 136–140, 1967
Branch, C. D., C. B. Sledge: Inflammatory lesions of the colon simulating neoplasms. Gastroenterology 28: 981–989, 1955
Braun, B. D.: The value of multiple barium studies. Amer. J. Roentgenol. 81: 661–674, 1959
Brenner, S. M., G. Annes, J. G. Parker: Tuberculous colitis simulating unspecific granulomatous disease of the colon. Amer. J. dig. Dis. 15: 85–92, 1970
Brombart, J. C., C. Hins: La polypose généralisée familiale du côlon. J. belge Radiol. 54: 45–51, 1971
Brombart, M., J. Massion: Radiologic differences between ileocecal tuberculosis and Crohn's disease. Amer. J. dig. Dis. 6: 589–603, 1961
Brooke, B. N.: Malignant change in ulcerative colitis. Dis. Colon Rect. 4: 393–398, 1961
Brooke, B. N.: Inflammatory disorders of colon. Dis. Colon Rect. 5: 138–144, 1962
Brooke, B. N.: The indication for emergency colectomy in ulcerative colitis. Dis. Colon Rect. 11: 85–90, 1968
Brown, D. C.: Changing concepts in diverticulosis of the colon. Amer. J. dig. Dis. 6: 791–797, 1961
Brown, D. C.: Changing concepts in diverticulosis of the colon. Geriatrics 16: 14–20, 1961
Brown, G. R.: A new approach to colon preparation for barium enema: Preliminary report. Univ. Mich. med. Bull. 27: 225–230, 1961
Brust, J. C. M.: Solitary adenomas of rectum and lower portion of sigmoid. Proc. Mayo Clin. 9: 625–631, 1934
Brust, J. C. M.: Polyps of the rectum and colon; their etiology, clinical significance and treatment. N. Y. St. J. Med. 42: 973–977, 1942
Buck, R. L.: Diverticulosis and diverticulitis. Review of cases at New Orleans Charity Hospital from 1950–1956. Discussion of complications and treatment. Dis. Colon Rect. 1: 205–208, 1958
Buckstein, J.: The digestive tract in roentgenology. Vol II. Lippincott, Philadelphia 1953
Buie, L.: Polypoid disease of the colon. J. Indian med. Ass. 30: 622–627, 1937
Bumm, R.: Die Divertikel des Dickdarms und ihre Komplikationen. Arch. klin. Chir. 174: 14–31, 1933
Burnikel, R. H., A. G. Schutte: Adenomatous polyps of the rectum and distal sigmoid; statistical analysis of 500 patients with polyps. Amer. J. Surg. 88: 378–383, 1954
Burns, F. J.: Bleeding diverticular disease of the colon. Sth. med. J. (Bgham, Ala.) 53: 312–314, 1960
Buskirk, W. C.: Polyps of the large bowel. Ann. Surg. 141: 234–239, 1955

Cabrera, A., J. Lega: Polyps of the colon and rectum in children. Amer. J. Surg. 100: 551–560, 1960
Carletti, C.: Il colon irritabile. Importanza dell' indagine radiologica ai fini della sua diagnosi. Minerva gastroent. 11: 55–70, 1965

Carrol, P.T.: Diverticula, diverticulosis and diverticulitis of the colon. Indications for operation and refinement of surgical technic. Dis. Colon Rect. 4: 88–102, 1961
Carrol, P.T., M.A.Anthony: Chronic ulcerative colitis in elderly patients. Dis. Colon Rect. 7: 226–235, 1964
Castleman, B., H.J.Krickstein: Do adenomatous polyps of the colon become malignant? New Engl. J. Med. 267: 469–475, 1962
Castro, A.F.: Adenomatous polyps of the rectum and colon in children. Clin. Proc. Child. Hosp. (Wash.) 11: 29–32, 1955
Castro, A.F.: The coexistence of diverticular disease and adenomatous polyps of the colon. Sth. med. J. 50: 1437–1440, 1957
Castro, A.F.: A reappraisal of the colonic polyp. Med. Ann. D. C. 32: 11–17, 1963
Castro, A.F., G.W.Ault, R.S.Smith: Adenomatous polyps of the colon and rectum. Surg. Gynec. Obstet. 92: 164–171, 1951
Cattell, R.B., N.W.Swinton: Diagnosis and treatment of sigmoid polyps. New Engl. J. Med. 222: 535–540, 1940
Cattell, R.B.: Surgical treatment of ulcerative colitis. Gastroenterology 10: 63–66, 1948
Cattell, R.B., N.W.Swinton: Significance and treatment of colonic and rectal polyps. Surg. Clin. N. Amer. 17: 857–863, 1937
Celio, A.: Zur Pathologie der chronischen stenosierenden Diverticulitis coli. Helv. chir. Acta 19: 93–118, 1952
Chaitin, H.: Evolution and diverticulosis and diverticulitis of the colon. Dis. Colon Rect. 9: 377–380, 1966
Chandhary, N., S.Truelove: Human colonic motility; A comparative study of normal subject, patients with ulcerative colitis and with the irritable colon syndrome. Gastroenterology 40: 1–36, 1961
Chapman, J.: Adenomatous polypi of the large intestine, incidence and distribution. Ann. Surg. 157: 223–226, 1963
Chrispin, A.R., J.K.Fry: The presacral space shown by barium enema. Brit. J. Radiol. 36: 319–322, 1963
Christie, A.C., F.O.Coe, A.O.Hampton, G.M.Wyat: The value of tannic acid enema post-evacuation roentgenograms in examination of colon. Amer. J. Roentgenol. 63: 657–664, 1950
Clements, N.C.: Diverticular disease of the colon as a cause of severe hemorrhage in the aged. Surg. Clin. N. Amer. 40: 933–944, 1960
Cobben, J.J.: The use of bisacodyl and the application of molecularly dispersed bisacodyl (dissolved in polyethylene glycol) in the cleansing enema and in the radiological contrast enema in the examination of the colon. Medica mundi 13: 76–88, 1969
Coffey, R.J., J.A.Bargen: Intestinal polyps: pathogenesis and relation to malignancy. Surg. Gynec Obstet. 69: 136–145, 1939
Coffey, R.J., F.J.Brinig: Symposium on diagnosis and treatment of premalignant conditions; polyps of large bowel. Surg. Clin. N. Amer. 30: 1749–1765, 1950
Cohen, W.N.: Roentgenographic evaluation of the rectal valves of Houston in the normal and in ulcerative colitis. Amer. J. Roentgenol. 104: 580–583, 1968
Cohen, S.E., B.L.Matthews: Dissecting diverticulitis of the colon. Surgery 28: 823–827, 1946
Cohen, S.E., J.R.Cunningham, H.Sneierson: The intramural diverticulum and dissecting diverticulitis. Arch. Surg. 75: 800–806, 1957
Colcock, B.P.: Ulcerative colitis. Indication for surgery and types of operation. Dis. Colon Rect. 3: 347–351, 1960
Colcock, B.P.: Carcinoma of the colon and rectum. Amer. Surg. 30: 6–8, 1964
Colcock, B.P., T.A.Lamphier: Endometriosis of the large and small intestine. Surgery 28: 997–1004, 1950
Colcock, B.P., R.E.Sass: Diverticulitis and carcinoma of the colon; differential diagnosis. Surg. Gynec. Obstet. 99: 627–633, 1954
Collins, V.P.: Time of occurrence of pulmonary metastasis from carcinoma of colon and rectum. Cancer 15: 387–395, 1962
Collins, V.P., R.K.Loeffler, H.Tivey: Observations on growth rates of human tumors. Amer. J. Roentgenol. 76: 988–1000, 1956
Colp, H.: Case of nonspecific granuloma of terminal ileum and cecum. Sth. Clin. N. Amer. 14: 443–449, 1934
Colvert, J.R., C.H.Brown: Rectal polyps; Diagnosis, 5 year follow-up and relation to carcinoma of the rectum. Amer. J. med. Sci. 215: 24–32, 1948
Connel, A.M.: Diverticular disease. Acta gastro-ent. belg. 30: 695–703, 1967
Cooper, W.L.: Sigmoidoscopic findings that suggest diverticulitis. Dis. Colon Rect. 1: 120–127, 1958
Cornes, J.S., M.Stecher: Primary Crohn's disease of colon and rectum. Gut 2: 189–201, 1961
Counsell, B.P., C.E.Dukes: Association of chronic ulcerative colitis and carcinoma of the colon and rectum. Brit, J. Surg. 39: 485–495, 1952
Cremin, B.J.: Lymphoid and other colon polyps in children. Ann. Radiol. 12: 199–204, 1969
Cremin, B.J., J.H.Louw: Polyps in the large bowel in children. Clin. Radiol. 21: 195–200, 1970
Crohn, B.B., A.A.Berg: Right-sided (regional) colitis. J. Amer. med. Ass. 110: 32–38, 1938
Crohn, B.B., L.Günzburg, G.D.Oppenheimer: Regional ileitis; pathological and clinical entity. J. Amer. med. Ass. 99: 1323–1329, 1932
Curry, C.: Polyps of the colon. J. Amer. osteopath. Ass. 54: 765–767, 1954

Daniels, V.C., E.H.Wood: Diverticulitis of cecum and ascending colon. J. Amer. med. Ass. 172: 519–524, 1960
David, V.C.: Pathology and treatment of bleeding polypoid tumors of large bowel. Surgery 100: 933–948, 1934
Deddish, M.R., R.E.Hertz: Symposium on early diagnosis of tumors of rectum and colon; colotomy and coloscopy in management of mucosal polyps and cancer of colon. Amer. J. Surg. 90: 846–849, 1955
Desai, M.G.: Varying radiological appearances in the terminal ileum associated with Crohn's disease. J. Fac. Radiol. (Lond.) 9: 99–105, 1958
Dick, A.P., F.R.Berridge, M.J.Grayson: The pathological basis of the radiological changes in ulcerative colitis. A study of cases treated by colectomy. Brit. J. Radiol. 32: 432–449, 1959
Diethelm, A.G., W.F.Nickel, G.E.Wantz: Ulcerative colitis in the elderly patient. Surg. Gynec. Obstet. 126: 1223–1229, 1968
Dietz, M.W.: Inflammatory colon stenoses. Radiology 93: 972, 1969
Diner, W.C., D.Dodd, O.E.Riggs: The value of bisacodyl Tannix (Clysodrast) in the radiological examination of the colon. Radiology 104: 49–51, 1972
Dockerty, M.: Pathologic aspects in the control of spread of colonic carcinoma. Proc. Mayo Clin. 33: 157–163, 1958
de Dombal, F.T., N.Geffen, A.Darmborough, G.Watkinson, J.C.Goligher: Radiological appearances of ulcerative colitis: an evaluation of their clinical significance. Gut. 9: 157–163, 1968
Dombrowski, H.: Die Röntgendiagnostik der entzündlichen Dickdarmerkrankungen. Internist (Berl.) 9: 343–352, 1968

Dombrowski, H.: A contribution to the roentgen diagnosis of granulomatous colitis (Crohn's disease) with a contribution concerning angiography. Radiologe 11: 264–273, 1971
Douglas, J.B.: The double contrast examination of the colon. Radiology 60: 490–495, 1953
Dreyfuss, J.R., M.L.Janover: Colon. In Golden's Diagnostic radiology. Williams and Wilkins, Baltimore 1969
Dukes, G.E.: Precancerous conditions of the colon and rectum. J. roy. Coll. Surg. (Edinb.) 3: 182–192, 1958
Dyer, N.H., A.M.Dawson: Diagnosis of Crohn's disease. A continuing source of error. Brit. med. J. 1: 735–737, 1970

Edling, N.P.G., O.A.Eklöf: A roentgenologic study of the course of ulcerative colitis. Acta radiol. (Stockh.) 54: 397–409, 1960
Edling, N.P.G., O.A.Eklöf: Distribution of malignancy in ulcerative colitis. Gastroenterology 41: 465–466, 1961
Edling, N.P.G., O.A.Eklöf: Radiologic findings and prognosis in ulcerative colitis. Acta chir. scand. 121: 299–308, 1961
Edling, N.P.G., O.A.Eklöf: The retrorectal soft-tissue space in ulcerative colitis: a roentgendiagnostic study. Radiology 80: 949–953, 1963
Edling, N.P.G., R.Lagercrantz, H.Rosenqvist: Roentgenologic findings in ulcerative colitis with malignant degeneration. Acta radiol. (Stockh.) 52: 123–128, 1959
Edwards, H.C.: Diverticula of the colon and vermiform appendix. Brit. J. Surg. 22: 88–107, 1934
Edwards, H.: Crohn's disease. An inquiry into its nature and consequences. Ann. roy. Coll. Surg. Engl. 44: 121–139, 1969
Egger, G., M.Härtel, F.Halter, J.Laissue: Non- gangrenous ischemic colitis: Clinical and radiological diagnosis. Fortschr. Röntgenstr. 115: 432–439, 1971
Ehrenpreis, T., N.O.Ericsson, L.Billing, R.Lagercrantz, U.Rudhe: Surgical treatment of ulcerative colitis in children. Acta paediat. (Uppsala) 49: 810–826, 1960
Ekelund, G.: On cancer and polyps of colon and rectum. Acta path. microbiol. scand. 59: 165–170, 1963
Ekelund, G.: On colorectal polyps and carcinoma with special reference to their interrelationship. Thesis, Studentlitteratur, Lund, 1974
Ekelund, G., C.Lindström, J.E.Rosengren: Roentgenologic signs and growth of early colorectal carcinomas. In preparation
Elmendorff, H.F., E.Marx, M.Hausmann: Sigmoiditis and diverticulitis. Langenbeck Arch. Chir. 312: 333–359, 1965
Engelbreth-Holm, J.: Ulcerative colitis after x-ray treatment for cancer of the uterus. Acta med. scand. 116: 308–321, 1944
Enquist, J.F.: The incidence and significance of polyps of the colon and rectum. Surgery 42: 681–688, 1957
Enquist, J.F., D.State: Rectal and colonic polyps. Surgery 32: 696–703, 1952
Enterline, H.T., G.W.Evans, R.Mercudo-Lugo, L.Miller, W.T.Fitts jr: Malignant potential of adenomas of colon and rectum. J. Amer. med. Ass. 179: 322–330, 1962
Erdman, J.F., J.H.Morris: Polyposis of the colon. Surg. Gynec. Obstet. 40: 460–468, 1925

Faccini, L.: Diverticula of the digestive tract. Ann. Radiol. diagn. (Bologna) 21: 157–257, 1949
Fahrländer, H.: Ulcerative colitis. A review based on 172 cases. Dtsch. med. Wschr. 91: 1953–1959, 1966
Farman, J., E.Betancourt, Z.M.Kilpatrick: The radiology of ischemic proctitis. Radiology 91: 302–307, 1968
Feldman, M.: Diverticulosis of the colon. In: Clinical Roentgenology of the digestive tract. 4th Ed. Williams and Wilkins, Baltimore 1957
Feldman, M., S.Morrison: Clinical evaluation of diverticulosis of the colon. Amer. J. dig. Dis. 16: 126–128, 1949
Felsen, J., W.Wolarsky: Chronic ulcerative colitis and carcinoma. Arch. int. Med. 84: 293–304, 1949
Fenger, C., K.Nyholm, E.Amdrup: Diverticulitis of the colon. Acta chir. scand., Suppl. 396: 114–120, 1969
Fennessy, J.J., M.B.Sparberg, J.B.Kirsner: Early roentgen manifestations of mild ulcerative colitis and proctitis. Radiology 87: 848–858, 1966
Fennessy, J.J., M.B.Sparberg, J.B.Kirsner: Radiological findings in carcinoma of the colon, complicating chronic ulcerative colitis. Gut 9: 383–397, 1968
Fernandez-Herlihy, L.: The articular manifestations of chronic ulcerative colitis. An analysis of 555 cases. New Engl. J. Med. 261: 259–263, 1959
Feyerter, F.: Zur Lehre von Polypenbildung im menschlichen Darm. Wien. med. Wschr. 79: 338–342, 1929
Fiebelkorn, H.J.: Die Reliefdarstellung des Dickdarmes mit "Unibaryt Rektal". Radiol. clin. (Basel) 23: 155–162, 1954
Fietz, H.: Differential diagnosis of Crohn's disease and tuberculosis of the intestine. Röntgen-Bl. 17: 91–98, 1964
Figiel, L.S., S.J.Figiel, A.Hennessy: Carcinoma of the colon. Incidence of error in the roentgen diagnosis. Amer. J. Gastroent. 40: 487–503, 1963
Figiel, L.S., S.J.Figiel, F.K.Wietersen: Is surgical removal of every colonic polyp necessary? Amer. J. Roentgenol. 88: 721–732, 1962
Figiel, L.S., S.J.Figiel, F.K.Wietersen: Conservative management of colonic polyps. Based on roentgenographic observations of growth. J. Mich. med. Soc. 62: 383–388, 1962
Figiel, S.J., L.S.Figiel, D.K.Rush: Study of colon by use of high-kilovoltage spot-compression technique. J. Amer. med. Ass. 166: 1269–1274, 1958
Finnley, J.M.T., D.H.Stone: The fallibility of roentgenograms in diagnosing lesions of the colon. Ann. Surg. 137: 674–686, 1953
Fischer, A.W.: Über eine neue röntgenologische Untersuchungsmethode des Dickdarms: Kombination von Kontrasteinlauf und Luftaufblähung. Klin. Wschr. 2: 1595–1598, 1923
Fischer, A.W.: Über die Röntgenuntersuchung des Dickdarms mit Hilfe einer Kombination von Lufteinblasung und Kontrasteinlauf. Langenbecks Arch. Chir. 134: 209–269, 1925
Fitts jr, W.T.: Adenomas of the colon and rectum. Their malignant potential. Amer. J. Surg. 101: 87–90, 1961
Fitzgibbon, G.: Polyps of the large intestine. Proc. Mayo Clin. 5: 157–159, 1930
Fitzgibbon, G., F.W.Rankin: Polyps of large intestine. Surg. Gynec. Obstet. 52: 1136–1150, 1931
Fleischner, F.G.: Diverticular disease and the irritable colon syndrome. In: Alimentary tract roentgenology, Sec. Ed. Mosby, St Louis 1967
Fleischner, F.G.: Diverticular disease of the colon. New observations and revised concepts. Gastroenterology 60: 316–324, 1971
Fleischner, F.G., P.Mandelstam: Roentgen observations of the ileostomy in patients with idiopathic ulcerative colitis. II: Ileostomy dysfunction. Radiology 70: 469–480, 1958
Fleischner, F.G., S.C.Ming, E.M.Henken: Revised concepts on diverticular disease of the colon. I: Diverticulosis: Emphasis on tissue derangement and its relation to the irritable colon syndrome. Radiology 83: 859–872, 1964

Fournier, A.M.: Use of double contrast in colon radiology. Marseille-med. 99: 1052–1053, 1962

Frech, K.: Die Rektographie. Fortschr. Röntgenstr. 78: 53–62, 1953

French, A.J., S.A.Vander: Idiopathic chronic ulcerative colitis and regional enterocolitis. Amer. J. Roentgenol. 74: 977–988, 1955

Friedland, G.W., G.J.Poole: False positive "Eccentric target sign" on barium air-contrast enema examination. Radiology 99: 67–68, 1971

Frimann-Dahl, J.: Radiological investigation in ulcerative colitis and Crohn's disease. T.Norsk Laegeforen Suppl. 919. 87: 880, 1967

Frye, T.R.: Villous adenoma of the sigmoid colon. Radiology 73: 71–75, 1959

Garland, H.: Discussion to Bell: General considerations. Radiology 55: 22–23, 1950

Garlock, J.H.: The surgical treatment of ulcerative colitis. Dis. Colon Rect. 2: 529–533, 1959

Garret, E.: The diagnosis of early cancer of the colon and rectum. Amer. J. dig. Dis. 17: 95–96, 1950

Geffen, N., N.Darnborough, F.T. de Dombal, G.Watkinson, J.C.Goligher: Radiological signs of ulcerative colitis: Assessment of their reliability by means of observer variation studies. Gut 9: 150–156, 1968

Geffroy, Y., J.Bourreille, R.Colin et al.: La réépithéliasation des lésions coliques de la maladie de Crohn. Etude anatomo-radiologique à propos de 5 cas d'ileocolite. Sem. Hôp. Paris 46: 2077–2083, 1970

Gelber, I., H.R.Hawthorne, A.Gelb: Carcinoma of the colon in ulcerative colitis. Gastroenterology 28: 836–841, 1955

Gershon-Cohen, J., H.Shay: Colon as studied by double contrast enema. Amer. J. Roentgenol. 27: 836–846, 1932

Gianturco, C.: Comparative value of various methods in the roentgenologic examination of colon. Illinois med. J. 71: 67–74, 1937

Gianturco, C.: High-voltage technic in the diagnosis of polypoid growths of the colon. Radiology 55: 27–29, 1950

Gianturco, C.: The radiological diagnosis of diverticula of the colon. Selected Papers Carle Hosp. Clin. 14: 19–20, 1961

Gianturco, C., G.Miller: Routine search for colonic polyps by high voltage radiography. Radiology 60: 496–499, 1953

Gianturco, C., G.Miller: Program for the detection of colonic and rectal polyps. J. Amer. med. Ass. 153: 1429–1430, 1953

Gilbert, R., S.Kadrnka: Examination of the mucosa of the digestive tract by means of umbrathor. Bull. Soc. Radiol. med. France 19: 101–104, 1931

Gilchrist, R.K., H.C.Breuhaus: X-ray and auxillary methods of diagnosing lower gastrointestinal lesions. Surg. Clin. N. Amer. 36: 161–168, 1956

Glay, A.: Toxic dilatation of the colon in the course of ulcerative colitis. Canad. Med. Ass. J. 88: 234–239, 1963

Goldberg, H.I.: Focal ulcerations of the colon in granulomatous colitis. Amer. J. Roentgenol. 101: 296–300, 1967

Goldberg, H.I., J.V.Carbone, A.R.Margulis: Roentgenographic reversibility of ulcerative colitis in children treated with steroid enemas. Amer. J. Roentgenol. 103: 365–379, 1968

Goldgraber, M.B.: Pseudopolyps in ulcerative colitis. Dis. Colon Rect. 8: 355–363, 1965

Goldgraber, M.B., J.B.Kirsner: Papilloma of the large intestine: a clinical-pathologic correlation. Gastroenterology 35: 36–49, 1958

Goldgraber, M.B., J.B.Kirsner, W.L.Palmer: The histopathology of chronic ulcerative colitis and its pathogenetic implications. Gastroenterology 38: 596–604, 1960

Goldgraber, M.B., E.M.Humphreys, J.B.Kirsner, W.L. Palmer: Carcinoma and ulcerative colitis. A clinical-pathologic study. Gastroenterology 36: 613–630, 1959

Goligher, J.C.: Primary excisional surgery in the treatment of ulcerative colitis. Ann. roy. Coll. Surg. Engl. 15: 316–325, 1954

Gombert, H.J.: Beitrag zum Thema: Innere Fisteln der Verdauungswege. Fortschr. Röntgenstr. 96: 692–694, 1962

Gordon, D.L., G.A.Hallenbeck, M.B.Dockerty, R.L. Kennedy, R.J.Jackman: Polyps of the colon in children. Arch. Surg. 75: 90–95, 1957

Goritzas, S., S.Benetatos: L'examen radiologique du colôn selon la méthode de Sölve Welin. J. Radiol. Électrol. 41: 779–790, 1960

Goulard, A.J., A.Hampton: Correlation of the clinical, pathological and roentgenological findings in diverticulitis. Amer. J. Roentgenol. 72: 213–221, 1954

Green, W.W.: Polyps of lower sigmoid and rectum. Ohio St. med. J. 37: 38–40, 1941

Groisser, V.W.: Granulomatous colitis. J. med. Soc. N.Y. 66: 608–611, 1969

Grout, J.L.A.: Symposium: diverticula of the alimentary tract. V. Diverticulosis and diverticulitis of the large intestine. Brit. J. Radiol. 22: 442–448, 1949

Haas, A., S.A.Ritter: Benign villous tumor. Amer. J. Proctol. 11: 201–211, 1960

Haenisch, G.F.: Die Röntgenuntersuchung bei Verengungen des Dickdarmes. Röntgenologische Frühdiagnose des Dickdarmkarzinoms. Münch. med. Wschr. 58: 2375–2381, 1911

Hahn, B., F.Doerr: Bemerkenswerte Komplikationen von Kolondivertikeln. Fortschr. Röntgenstr. 108: 643–648, 1968

Hall, G.H.: Polypoid adenomas of rectum and colon in children. Lancet 70: 440–441, 1950

Hamilton, J.B.: Use of tannic acid in barium enemas. Amer. J. Roentgenol. 56: 101–103, 1946

Hammer, B., P.Ashurst, J.Naish: Disease associated with ulcerative colitis and Crohn's disease Gut 9: 17–21, 1968

Hammer, G.: Die Röntgendiagnose der Darmtuberkulose. Fortschr. Röntgenstr. 36: 519–142, 1927

Hanley, P.H., M.O.Hines, J.E.Ray, F.McPherson, W.A. Hibbert: Villous tumors, experience with 163 patients. Sth. med. (Bgham, Ala.) J. 55: 233–238, 1962

Hardy, T.L., E.Bulmer: Ulcerative colitis; survey of 95 cases. Brit. med. J. 2: 812–815, 1933

Harper, R.A.K., J.H.L.Conway-Hughes: The tannic acid barium enema in colonic investigation. J. Fac. Radiol. (Lond.) 2: 168–176, 1950

Harris, J.W.: Polyps of rectum in children. Amer. J. Surg. 86: 577–581, 1953

Hartweg, H., H.Fahrländer: Die Crohnsche Erkrankung des Dickdarmes. Fortschr. Röntgenstr. 115: 439–456, 1971

Hartwell, J.A., R.L.Cecil: Intestinal diverticula: pathological and clinical study. Amer. J. med. Sci. 140: 174–203, 1910

Hawk, W.A., R.B.Turnbull jr, P.T.Schofield: Nonspecific ulcerative colitis. Surgery 66: 953–964, 1969

Hawkes, S.Z., R.K.Shields: Adenomatosis versus pseudopolyposis of large bowel. Bull. U.S. Army med. Dep. 6: 302–310, 1946

Heald, R.J., J.E.Ray: Bleeding from diverticula of the colon. Dis. Colon Rect. 14: 420–427, 1971

Heilbrun, N., C. Bernstein: Difficulties in the roentgen diagnosis of cecal tumors. Amer. J. Roentgenol. 87: 693–705, 1962
Helwig, E. B.: Benign tumors of the large intestine. Incidence and distribution. Surg. Gynec. Obstet. 76: 419–426, 1943
Helwig, E. B.: Adenomas of large intestine in children. Amer. J. Dis. Childh. 72: 289–295, 1946
Helwig, E. B.: Evolution of adenomas of the large intestine and their relation to carcinoma. Surg. Gynec. Obstet. 84: 36–49, 1947
Helwig, E. B.: Adenomas and the pathogenesis of cancer of the colon and rectum. Dis. Colon Rect. 2: 5–17, 1959
Helwig, F. C.: The association of benign and malignant polyps of the large intestine. Dis. Colon Rect. 3: 343–346, 1960
Hemmati, A.: Toxic dilatation of the colon in ulcerative colitis. Fortschr. Röntgenstr. 102: 265–267, 1965
Henshall, G. K.: Villous tumors of the large bowel and presentation of an unusual case. Amer. J. Roentgenol. 84: 1105–1113, 1960
Herbert, W. W.: Dynamic or disappearing diverticula of the colon. Radiology 91: 508–513, 1968
Hersch, R. A., A. D. Schwabe: Left hydronephrosis as complication of acute sigmoid diverticulitis. Gastroenterology 45: 269–273, 1963
Hertzberg, J.: Regional enteritis (Crohn's disease) localized to the colon. T. Norsk Laegeforen Suppl. 87: 914–916, 1967
Hettler, M.: Zur Technik der Doppelkontrastdarstellung des Dickdarmes. Radiologe 2: 115–124, 1962
Hildebrand, H.: Über den diagnostischen Wert der Röntgenstrahlen in der inneren Medizin. Münch. med. Wschr. 48: 2008–2012, 1901
Hines, M. O., P. H. Hanley, J. E. Ray, M. Bralliar: Villous tumors of the colon and rectum. Dis. Colon Rect. 1: 128–131, 1958
Hines, M. O., P. H. Hanley, J. E. Ray, B. M. Rush: Polyps of the colon and rectum in children. Experience with 27 cases. Dis. Colon Rect. 2: 161–165, 1959
Hinton, J. W.: Treatment of diverticulitis of the large intestine and its complications. Dis. Colon Rect. 2: 426–437, 1959
Hodges, F. M.: The roentgen ray in the diagnosis of mucous colitis. Radiology 13: 383–387, 1929
Hodges, P. C.: Roentgen examination of the colon. J. Amer. med. Ass. 153: 1417–1421, 1953
Hodgson, J. R., R. L. J. Kennedy: The roentgenologic aspects of chronic ulcerative colitis in children. Radiology 65: 671–679, 1955
Hodgson, J. R., G. Sauer: The roentgenologic features of carcinoma in chronic ulcerative colitis. Amer. J. Roentgenol. 86: 91–96, 1961
Hoerner, M. T.: Carcinoma of the colon and rectum in persons under twenty years of age. Amer. J. Surg. 96: 47-53, 1958
Holgersen, L. O., R. E. Miller, H. A. Zintel: Juvenile polyps of the colon. Surgery 69: 288–293, 1971
Hoon, J. R., M. B. Dockerty, J. Pemberton: Collective review; ileocecal tuberculosis including a comparison of this disease with nonspecific regional enterocolitis and noncaseous tuberculated enterocolitis. Internat. Abstr. Surg. 60: 417–440, 1950
Horner, J. L.: Natural history of diverticulosis of the colon. Amer. J. dig. Dis. 3: 343–350, 1958
Horrilleno, E. G., C. Eckert, L. V. Ackerman: Polyps of the rectum and colon in children. Cancer 10: 1210–1220, 1957
Hughes, E. S. R.: Acute ulcerative colitis. Dis. Colon rect. 4: 3–16, 1961
Hughes, J. R., R. T. Jenkins, D. E. Sturdy: Single polyp of the large intestine in childhood. Arch. Dis. Childh. 31: 124–125, 1956
Hultborn, K. A.: Cancer of the colon and rectum. Acta chir. scand., Suppl. 172: 1–190, 1952
Hultborn, K. A.: The causal relationship between benign epithelial tumors and adenocarcinomas of the colon and rectum. Acta radiol. (Stockh.), Suppl. 113: 1–71, 1954
Hultborn, K. A., O. Morales, R. Romanus: The so-called shelf tumor of the rectum. Acta radiol. (Stockh.), Suppl. 124: 1–46, 1955
Hultén, J.: Diverticula of the veriform appendix, right colon and terminal ileum. Acta chir. scand. 124: 340–347, 1962
Hummel, R.: Differentialdiagnostische Schwierigkeiten zwischen Divertikulose des Dickdarmes und Neubildung. Med. Welt (Berlin) 9: 1657–1658, 1935

Jackman, K. V., E. W. Douglas: Crohn's disease of the large bowel. Surgery 66: 980–985, 1969
Jackman, R. J., C. W. Mayo: The adenoma-carcinoma sequence in cancer of the colon. Surg. Gynec. Obstet. 93: 327–330, 1951
Jacobs, E.: Changing concepts of diverticular disease of the colon. Dis. Colon Rect. 14: 29–31, 1971
Jalan, K. N., R. J. Walker, R. J. Prescott, S. T. G. Butterworth, A. N. Smith, W. Sircus: Faecal stasis and diverticular disease in ulcerative colitis. Gut 11: 688–696, 1970
Janowitz, H. D.: Notes on the panel on granulomatous colitis at the annual meeting of the american gastroenterologic association Chicago. Gastroenterology 51: 588–591, 1966
Janowitz, H. D., A. E. Lindner, R. H. Marshak: Granulomatous colitis. Crohn's disease of the colon. J. Amer. med. Ass. 191: 825–828, 1965
Jarre, H. A., S. J. Figiel: Refinements in radiologic diagnosis of colonic disease. In Rajewsky, B. editor, Proceedings of Ninth International Congress of Radiology, Münich 1959, Vol. I. Thieme, Stuttgart 1961
Jeanmart, L., A. Bremer, J. Dagnelie, V. et R. Capon: Les tumeurs villeuses du côlon. J. belge Radiol. 54: 73–81, 1971
Jensen, G. L.: Massive hemorrhage from diverticulosis of the colon. Amer. J. Surg. 95: 813–817, 1958
Jew jr, E. W., S. P. Harbison: Resection for diverticular disease of the sigmoid colon. Arch. Surg. 81: 435–443, 1960
Johnson, T. M., T. G. Orr: Carcinoma of colon, secondary to chronic ulcerative colitis. Amer. J. dig. Dis. 15: 21–23, 1948
Johnstone, A. S.: Symposium on diverticula of the alimentary tract. Brit. J. Radiol. 22: 415–418, 1949
Jones, H. H., H. S. Kaplan, F. Windholz: Air-contrast colon examination with colloidal barium. Radiology 56: 561–566, 1951
Jones, J. H.: Colonic cancer and Crohn's disease. Gut 10: 651–654, 1969
Jones, J. H., J. E. Lennard-Jones, A. C. Young: Reversibility of radiological appearance during clinical improvement in colonic Crohn's disease. Gut 10: 738–743, 1969
Judd jr, E. S., J. C. Carlisle: Polyps of colon. Arch. Surg. 67: 353–362, 1953
Judd, E. S., M. P. Smith: Present trends in surgical treatment of diverticulitis. Surg. Clin. N. America 37: 1019–1027, 1957

Kalil, T. H., L. L. Robbins: Early roentgenologic changes in idiopathic ulcerative colitis. Radiology 53: 1–10, 1949
Kalkbrenner, H.: Über eine neue röntgenologische Untersuchungsmethode des Dickdarmes: die Darstellung des Schleimhautreliefs mit Umbrathor. Fortschr. Röntgenstr. 38: 325–332, 1928

Kaye, J.I., D.G.Bragg: Unusual roentgenologic and clinicopathologic features of villous adenomas of the colon. Radiology 91: 799–806, 1968
Keely, F., V.K.Gohel, P.J.Hodes: A roentgenologic remission in ulcerative colitis. Amer. J. Roentgenol. 86: 906–910, 1961
Keith, A.: Diverticula of the alimentary tract of congenital or oscene origin. Brit. med. J. 1: 376–380, 1910
Kendig, T.A.: Personal reference (Long Beach, Calif.)
Kennedy, R.: Polyps of rectum and colon in infants and children. Amer. J. Dis. Child. 62: 481–488, 1941
Kennedy, R.L.J., C.F.Dixon, H.M.Weber: Polypoid lesions of the colon of children. Surg. Gynec. Obstet. 77: 639–644, 1943
Kent, K.H., H.J.Raszkowski: Colon lesions masqueradens as small bowel obstruction on the plain roentgenogram of the abdomen. Amer. J. Roentgenol. 88: 671–676, 1962
Kerr, J.G.: Polyposis of the colon in chlidren. Amer. J. Surg. 76: 667–670, 1948
Khubchadani, I., H.E.Bacon: Malignant degeneration in ulcerative colitis. Dis. Colon Rect. 8: 201–204, 1965
King, R.C., A.E.Lindner, H.M.Pollard: Chronic ulcerative colitis in childhood: a follow-up study. Arch. Dis. Childh. 34: 257–261, 1959
Klein, R.R., R.A.Scarborough: Diagnosis and treatment of adenomatous polyps of colon. Arch. Surg. 65: 65–71, 1952
Knothe, W.: Röntgenstudien am Schleimhautrelief des normalen und kranken Dickdarmes. Fortschr. Röntgenstr. 36: 55–56, 1927
Knox, W.G., R.E.Miller, C.F.Begg, H.A.Zintel: Juvenile polyps of the colon. A clinicopathologic analysis of 75 polyps in 43 patients. Surgery 48: 201–210, 1960
Köhler, R.: The incidence of colonic diverticulosis in Finland and Sweden. Acta chir. scand. 126: 148–155, 1963
Kolodny, M.: Reversible right colonic strictures in chronic ulcerative colitis. Radiology 97: 83–84, 1970
Koppel, M., J.C.Bailar, F.L.Weakly, M.B.Shimkin: Incidence of cancer in colon and rectum among polypfree patients. Dis. Colon Rect. 5: 349–355, 1962
Korsgaard, B., M.Holm, M.Katznelson: The relation between radiological changes and clinical state in ulcerative colitis. Scand. J. Gastroent. 4: 297–303, 1969
Kraemer, M., L.H.Siegel: Diverticulitis coli with perforation, resembling ileitis. Gastroenterology 11: 538–543, 1948
Kratzer, G.L., J.H.Wadie: Acute fulminating ulcerative colitis. Dis. Colon Rect. 4: 424-428, 1961
Kroening, P.M.: Sigmoido-ileal fistulas as a complication of diverticulitis. Amer. J. Roentgenol. 96: 323–325, 1966
Kutting, J.: Die Rektographie. Fortschr. Röntgenstr. 79: 761–763, 1953
Kühne, H.: Die Divertikulose des Dickdarms und ihre Komplikationen. Zbl. Chir. 83: 801–815, 1958
Kühne, H., H.Bellman: Fatal complications of colonic diverticulosis. Zbl. Chir. 93: 778–782, 1968

Lackey, R.S.: Considerations of roentgenographic changes associated with ulcerative colitis. N. Carolina med. J. 24: 504–507, 1963
Lagercrantz, R.: Follow-up investigation of children with ulcerative colitis: with special reference to indications for surgical therapy. Acta paediat. (Uppsala) 44: 302–317, 1955
Laimon, H., P.Cohn: Diverticulitis of the coecum. A report of 8 cases. Amer. J. Surg. 103: 146–149, 1962
Lavaurs, G., M.Carcasonne, J.David: Etude radiologique des tumeurs inflammatoirs du côlon droit. Ann. Radiol. 5: 295–308, 1962
Lavaurs, G., M.Carcasonne, A.Zumino: Sigmoiditis simulating tumor. Ann. Radiol. 5: 667–682, 1962
LeBlan, L.J., G.L.Krause: Adenomatous polyps of large bowel. Missouri Med. 50: 925–928, 1953
Ledoux-Lebard, R., J.Garcia-Calderon: Les techniques d'examen de la muqueuse du gros intestine. J. Radiol. Électrol. 17: 429–464, 1933
Lehman, K.: Diverticulitis coli, with special regard to treatment and prognosis. Acta chir. scand., Suppl. 357: 206–208, 1966
Lennard-Jones, J.E., H.E.Lockhart-Mummery, B.C. Morson: Clinical and pathological differentiation of Crohn's disease and proctitis. Gastroenterology 54: 1162–1170, 1968
Levene, G.: A new method for the roentgenologic study of the rectum. Surgery 25: 68–75, 1949
Levene, G., N.C.Veale: The inadequacy of routine barium enema for roentgenologic examination of rectum. Amer. J. dig. Dis. 18: 175–181, 1951
Liguory, C., F.Bouskela, Conte-Marti et al: Etudes radioloque et anatomique comparées de la colite ulcéreuse. Sem. Hôp. Paris 44: 1572–1585, 1968
Lindner, A.E., R.C.King, R.J.Bolt: Chronic ulcerative colitis. A clinical appraisal and followup study. Gastroenterology 39: 153–160, 1960
Lockhart-Mummery, H.E.: Symposium on ulcerative colitis. Pathology of ulcerative colitis. Dis. Colon Rect. 3: 368–369, 1960
Lockhart-Mummery, H.E.: Pathologic lesions of the anal region associated with Crohn's disease. Dis. Colon Rect. 8: 399–401, 1965
Lockhart-Mummery, H.E., B.C.Morson: Crohn's disease (regional enteritis) of the large intestine and its distinction from ulcerative colitis. Gut 1: 87–105, 1960
Lockhart-Mummery, J.P.: Causation and treatment of multiple adenomatosis of the colon. Ann. Surg. 99: 178–184, 1934
Lockhart-Mummery, J.P., H.L.Hodgson: Observations on diverticula of colon and their sequelae. Brit. med. J. 1: 525–527, 1931
deLor, C.J.: The irritable bowel syndrome. Amer. J. Gastroent. 47: 427–434, 1967
Lörinc, P., F.Brahme: Perforation of the colon during examination by the double contrast method. Gastroenterology 37: 770–773, 1959
Lucke, H.H., K.E.Hodge, N.L.Patt: Fatal liver damage after barium enemas containing tannic acid. Canad. med. Ass. J. 89: 1111–1114, 1963
Lumb, G., R.H.B.Protheroe, G.S.Ramsay: Ulcerative colitis with dilatation of the colon. Brit. J. Surg. 43: 182–188, 1955
Lumsden, K., S.C.Truelove: Radiology of the digestive system. Blackwell, Oxford 1965 pp. 332–340
Lumsden, K., N.A.Chaudhary, S.C.Truelove: The irritable colon syndrome. Clin. Radiol. 14: 54–63, 1965

McAlister, W.H., M.S.Anderson, G.R.Bloomberg, A.R. Margulis: Lethal effects of tannic acid in the barium enema. (Reports of three fatalities and experimental studies). Radiology 80: 765–773, 1963
McCarthy, J.D., J.G.Picazo: Diverticulitis – A case reflecting upon pathogenesis. Dis. Colon Rect. 12: 451–452, 1969
McConnel, F., J.Hanelin, L.A.Robbins: Plain film diagnosis of fulminating ulcerative colitis. Radiology 71: 674–682, 1958
McCormick, N.A.: Diagnosis of early cancer of the large bowel and rectum. Canad med. Ass. J. 64: 403–409, 1951
McGowern, V.J.: The pathology of ulcerative colitis. J. Coll. Radiol. Aust. 7: 168–170, 1963

McGregor, R.A., H.E.Bacon: Diverticular disease of the colon. Dis. Colon Rect. 1: 197–204, 1958
McInerny, G.T., W.G.Sauer, A.H.Baggenstoss, J.H. Hodgson: Fulminating ulcerative colitis with marked colonic dilatation: a clinopathologic study. Gastroenterology 42: 244–257, 1962
McLanahan, S., G.P.Grove, R.F.Kieffer jr: Conservative surgical management for certain rectal adenomas showing malignant change. J. Amer. med. Ass. 141: 822–826, 1949
McLaren, J.W., J.B.King, W.A.Copland: Preliminary observations on Veripaque, a colonic actuator for use with barium enemata. Brit. J. Radiol. 28: 285–294, 1955
McLaren, J.W., J.B.King, W.A.Copland: Further observations on the use of dihydroxyphenylisatin in barium enemata. Brit. J. Radiol. 30: 223–224, 1957
McMillan, F.L., R.M.Potter: Small lesions of colon. Arch. Surg. 64: 686–696, 1952
Maingot, G., R.Sarasin, H.Duclos: Diverticulose et diverticulite des côlons. Bull. Soc. radiol. méd. France 22: 488–492, 1934
Marcus, R., J.Watt: The "pre-diverticular state". Its relationship to diverticula in the anti-mesenteric intertaenia area of the pelvic colon. Brit. J. Surg. 51: 676–682, 1964
Marcus, R., J.Watt: The radiological appearance of diverticula in the antimesenteric intertaenia area of the pelvic colon. Clin. Radiol. 16: 87–92, 1965
Marganoff, H.: Anorectal lesions associated with granulomatous colitis. Dis. Colon Rect. 9: 49–57, 1966
Margulis, A.R.: Radiology of ulcerating colitis. Radiology 105: 251–263, 1972
Margulis, A.R., H.I.Goldberg: The current state of radiologic technique in the examination of the colon: a survey. Radiol. Clin. N. America 7: 27–42, 1969
Margulis, A.R., H.I.Goldberg, T.L.Lawson et al.: The overlapping spectrum of ulcerative and granulomatous colitis; a roentgenographic-pathologic study. Amer. J. Roentgenol. 113: 325–334, 1971
Marques, P., H.Pons: Radiology of diverticulosis of the colon. Differential diagnosis. Arch. Mal. Appar. dig. 40: 1409–1418, 1971
Marshak, R.H.: Diverticulitis with abscess formation and vaginal fistula. Radiology 50: 92–95, 1948
Marshak, R.H.: The pedunculated adenomatous polyp. Amer. J. dig. Dis. 10: 958–967, 1965
Marshak, R.H.: Roentgen features of granulomatous colitis. Bull. N.Y. Acad. Med. 43: 910–923, 1967
Marshak, R.H., J.Eliasoph: Inflammatory lesions of the small bowel secondary to colonic diverticulitis. Amer. J. dig. Dis. 6: 423–428, 1961
Marshak, R.H., A.E.Lindner: Granulomatous colitis. Sem. Roentgenol. 3: 27–61, 1968
Marshak, R.H., A.E.Lindner: The radiology corner. Amer. J. Gastroent. 53: 478–481, 1970
Marshak, R.H., C.Bloch, B.S.Wolf: The roentgen findings in strictures of the colon associated with ulcerative and granulomatous colitis. Amer. J. Roentgenol. 90: 709–716, 1963
Marshak, R.H., A.E.Lindner, H.D.Janowitz: Granulomatous ileocolitis. Gut 7: 258–264, 1966
Marshak, R.H., J.E.Moseley, B.S.Wolf: The roentgen findings in familial polyposis with special emphasis on differential diagnosis. Radiology 80: 374–382, 1963
Marshak, R.H., B.S.Wolf, J.Eliasoph: Segmental colitis. Radiology 73: 707–716, 1959
Marshak, R.H., B.I.Korelitz, S.H.Klein, B.S.Wolf, H.D.Janowitz: Toxic dilatation of the colon in the course of ulcerative colitis. Gastroenterology 38: 165–180, 1960
Martin jr., W.J.: Polypoid lesions of the colon and rectum. (Malignant degeneration). Trans. Amer. proctol. Soc. 40: 176–183, 1939
Massik, P., F.E.Wheatly: The recognition of air in diverticula of the colon as a diagnostic aid. Radiology 64: 417–419, 1955
Masson, J.: Le diagnostic radiologique de la diverticulite du colôn. Rev. méd. Suisse rom. 56: 154–176, 1936
Maurer, H.J.: Das inkomplette Dickdarmdivertikel. Dtsch. med. Wschr. 91: 1786–1787, 1966
Maurer, H.J.: Diagnosis and clinical findings of the incomplete diverticulum of the colon. Röntgen-Bl. 21: 90–95, 1968
Mayo, W.J.: Diverticulitis of the sigmoid. Brit. med. J. 2: 574–576, 1929
Mayo, C.W., C.P.Blunt: Surgical management of the complications of diverticulitis of the large intestine. Surg. Clin. N. America 30: 1005–1012, 1950
Meadows, T.R., J.C.Batsakis: Histopathological spectrum of regional enteritis. Arch. Surg. 87: 976–982, 1963
Meier, C.D., H.J.Burhenne: Indirect roentgen changes in the colon produced by regional enteritis. Radiology 80: 50–56, 1963
Meyers, S.G., P.E.Ruble, L.B.Ashley: Clinical course of regional ileitis. Amer. J. dig. Dis. 4: 341–351, 1959
Miangolarra, C.J.: Diverticulitis of the right colon: an important surgical problem. Ann. Surg. 153: 861–870, 1961
Miller, W.B., B.Felson: Diverticulitis of the terminal ileum. Amer. J. Roentgenol. 96: 361–365, 1966
Ming, S.C., F.G.Fleischner: Diverticulitis of the sigmoid colon. Reappraisal of the pathology and pathogenesis. Surgery 58: 627–633, 1965
Mirvish, L.: Diverticulitis of the coecum. Clin. Proc. 5: 354–359, 1946
Moller, C., L.Stjernvull: Ischaemic colitis. Acta chir. scand. 137: 75–79, 1971
Monat, H.A.: Ulcerative colitis. Amer. J. Proctol. 7: 402–405, 1956
Moreton, R.D.: Double contrast examination of the colon with special emphasis on studies of the sigmoid. Radiology 60: 510–517, 1953
Moreton, R.D., C.W.Yates: Roentgenologic study of the colon: value of the double contrast enema. Tex. St. J. Med. 45: 157–163, 1949
Moreton, R.D., C.W.Yates: The double contrast study of the colon; a comparative study of barium sulfate preparation. Radiology 54: 541–547, 1950
Moreton, R.D., E.M.Cooper, E.F.Foegelle: A simple one-stage method of double-contrast study of the colon. Radiology 56: 214–221, 1951
Moreton, R.D., C.A.Stevenson, C.W.Yates: Fictitious polyps as seen in double-contrast studies of the colon. Radiology 53: 386–393, 1949
Morson, B.C.: The muscle abnormality in diverticular disease of the sigmoid colon. Brit. J. Radiol. 36: 385–392, 1962
Morson, B.C.: Factors influencing the prognosis of early cancer of the rectum. Proc. roy. Soc. Med. 59: 607–608, 1966
Morson, B.C.: Histopathology of Crohn's disease. Proc. roy. Soc. Med. 61: 79–81, 1968
Morson, B.C., H.E.Lockhart-Mummery: Anal lesions in Crohn's disease. Lancet 2: 1122–1131, 1959
Morton, D.L., L.Goldman: Differential diagnosis of diverticulitis and carcinoma of the sigmoid colon. Amer. J. Surg. 103: 55–61, 1962
Morton, J.J.: Diverticulitis and carcinoma of the sigmoid. Surgery 32: 765–783, 1952
Morton, P.C.: Adenomas of colon and rectum: Diagnosis and treatment in relation to cancer prevention. Ann. Surg. 138: 92–98, 1953
Mosbech, J.: Mortality from ulcerative colitis in Denmark. Gastroenterology 39: 690–694, 1960

Mosely, J.E., R.H.Marshak, B.S.Wolf: Regional enteritis in children. Amer. J. Roentgenol. 84: 532–539, 1960
Mottram, J.C.: On the origin of tar tumors in mice, whether from single cells or many cells. J. Path. Bact. 40: 407–414, 1935
Mussgnug, G., H.Wegener, J. Portmann: Pseudocarcinomatous tumors of the colon in diverticulitis. Fortschr. Röntgenstr. 99: 72–77, 1963
De Muth jr, W.E., P.J.Cherney, W.T.Fitts jr: Adenomatous polyps of the colon and rectum; a challenge in cancer prophylaxis. Surg. Gynec. Obstet. 94: 195–199 1952
Myers, T.B., H.E.Bacon: Adenomas of the colon and rectum. Dis. Colon Rect. 3: 523–532, 1960

Nathan, M.H., V.P.Collins, R.A.Adams: Differentiation of benign and malignant pulmonary nodules by growth rate. Radiology 79: 221–231, 1962
Naud, A.: Observation clinique et radiologique d'un cas de maladie de Crohn chez enfant. J. Radiol. Électrol. 44: 195–197, 1963
Neschis, M., S.S.Siegelman, J.G.Parker: Diagnosis and management of the megacolon of ulcerative colitis. Gastroenterology 55: 251–259, 1968
Neuman, H.W., J.A.Bargen, E.S.Judd jr: Clinical study of 201 cases of regional (segmental) colitis. Surg. Gynec. Obstet. 99: 563–571, 1954
Nissenbaum, J., A.J.Sparks, G.R.Ellison: Cecal diverticulum. Report of a case diagnosed by roentgen ray and surgically proved: review of the original literature. Amer. J. Roentgenol. 73: 596–605, 1955
Nolan, D.J., W.J.Norman, G.R.Airth: Traction diverticula of the colon. Clin. Radiol. 22: 458–461, 1971
Noveroske, R.J.: Intracolonic pressures during barium enema examination. Amer. J. Roentgenol. 91: 852–863, 1964

Oberhelman, H.A.: Sources of error in treatment of sigmoid diverticulitis. Surg. Clin. N. America 38: 257–266, 1958
Ochsner, S.F.: Diverticulosis of the appendix. Radiology 77: 100–102, 1961
Oestern, H.F., H.W.Schreiber: Über die Pathologie und Klinik der Divertikulose und Divertikulitis. Langenbecks Arch. Chir. 286: 411–430, 1958
Olson, R.W., J.R.Hodgson, W.G.Sauer: The roentgen diagnosis of diverticulitis. Radiology 80: 392–398, 1963
Oppenheimer, A., G.W.Saleeby: Proctography; roentgenologic studies of rectum and sigmoid. Surg. Gynec. Obstet. 69: 83–93, 1939
Ortmayer, M.: Small polyps of rectum and lower sigmoid. Their relationship to carcinoma of the distal colon. J. Am. M.Women's A. 5: 217–221, 1950
Ortmayer, M.: Carcinoma in small polyps of the distal colon: a sigmoidoscopic and histologic study. Gastroenterology 31: 404–412, 1956
Otani, S., I.Snapper: An incidence of carcinoma in chronic ulcerative colitis. J. Mt. Sinai Hosp. 19: 275–288, 1952

Packard, R.S.: Non-specific colitis. J. Coll. Radiol. Aust. 7: 159–162, 1963
Painter, N.S.: Diverticular disease. Tutorials in Postgrad. Med. 1: 201–217, 1969
Pansdorf, H.: Die Röntgendiagnostik der entzündlichen Dickdarmerkrankungen und ihre Abgrenzung gegenüber dem Carcinom. Röntgenpraxis 2: 732–740, 1930
Papp, J.P., H.M.Pollard: Toxic dilatation of the colon in granulomatous colitis. Report of 2 cases. Amer. J. dig. Dis. 15: 1105–1113, 1970
Parks, T.G., A.M.Connell: The outcome in 455 patients admitted for treatment of diverticular disease of the colon. Brit. J. Surg. 57: 775–778, 1970
Parks, T.G., A.M.Connell, A.D.Gough, J.O.Y.Cole: Limitations of radiology in the differentiation of diverticulitis and diverticulosis of the colon. Brit. med. J. 2: 136–138, 1970
van Patter, W.N. and others: Regional enteritis. Gastroenterology 26: 347–350, 1954
Patterson, H.A.: Diverticulitis of the colon. Amer. J. Gastroent. 44: 346–356, 1965
Paulino, F., A.Roselli, U.Martins: Pathology of diverticular disease of the colon. Surgery 69: 63–69, 1971
Peale, A.R.: Pathologic differentiation between regional enteritis and ulcerative colitis. Dis. Colon Rect. 5: 184–192, 1962
Peck, D.A., R.Labat, V.C.Waite: Diverticular disease of the right colon. Dis. Colon Rect. 11: 49–54, 1968
de Peister, F.A., R.K.Gilchrist: Symposium on function and disease of anorectum and colon: pathology of cancer of colon and rectum; classification and models of spread. Surg. Clin. N. Amer. 35: 1295–1305, 1955
Perret, A.D., S.C.Truelove, G.R.Massarella: Crohn's disease and carcinoma of the colon. Brit. med. J. 2: 466–468, 1968
Peskin, G.W., A.V.O.Davis: Acute fulminating ulcerative colitis with colonic distention. Surg. Gynec. Obstet. 110: 269–276, 1960
Phillips, R.B.: Polyps of colon and rectum; their association with cancer. Milit. Surg. 88: 258–264, 1941
Phillips, W.M., W.H.Remine, O.H.Beahrs, H.H.Scudamore: Benign lesions of the cecum simulating carcinoma. J. Amer. med. Ass. 172: 1465–1468, 1960
Pickens jr, D.R., J.L.Farringer: Familial polyposis and the spontaneous regression of polyps. Amer. Surg. 35: 361–365, 1969
Platt, J.W., B.E.Schlesinger, P.E.Benson: Ulcerative colitis in childhood: a study of its natural history. Quart. J. Med. 29: 257–277, 1960
Polgar, F.: Contrast enema in lateral recumbency; aimed gas filling of the colon. Radiology 53: 49–58, 1949
Poppel, M.H., S.L.Beranbaum: The indenture sign in acute exudative colitis. Amer. J. dig. Dis. 2: 382–386, 1957
Portes, C., J.D.Majarakis: Proctosigmoidoscopyincidence of polyps in 50,000 examinations. J. Amer. med. Ass. 163: 411–413, 1957
Potter, R.M.: Dilute contrast media in diagnosis of lesions of the colon. Radiology 60: 500–509, 1953
Prévôt, R.: Grundriß der Röntgenologie des Magen-Darm-Kanals. Nölke, Hamburg 1948
Prévôt, R.: Zur Röntgenologie der regionalen Enteritis. Gastroenterologia (Basel) 95: 268–280, 1961
Prévôt, R.: Zur Röntgendiagnostik der Ileocolitis (Brooke-Cooke). Radiologe 4: 377–380, 1946
Prévôt, R., M.A.Lassrich: Röntgendiagnostik des Magen-Darmkanals. Thieme, Stuttgart 1955

Quinn, W.C.: Gross hemorrhage from presumed diverticular disease of the colon: results of treatment in 103 patients. Ann. Surg. 153: 851–860, 1961

Rankin, F.W., A.S.Graham: Cancer of colon and rectum. Thomas, Springfield 1939
Rappaport, H., F.H.Burgoyne, H.F.Smetana: Pathology of regional enteritis. Milit. Surg. 109: 463–502, 1951
Ravdin, I.S.: Polyps of the colon – significance and management. J. nat. med. Ass. (N.Y.) 52: 387–392, 1960
Reeves, B.F., H.C.Carlson, M.B.Dockerty: Segmental ulcerative colitis versus segmental Crohn's disease of the colon. A roentgenographic and pathologic study. Amer. J. Roentgenol. 99: 24–34, 1967

Reeves, C.D., L.Raterman, H.H.Belding: Surgical treatment of diverticulitis of the colon. Amer. Surg. 35: 203–209, 1969
Reichman, H.R., G.H.Walker: Diverticulitis of the colon. Sth. med. J. (Bghm, Ala.) 53: 585–589, 1960
Reifferscheid, M.: Das Spätschicksal des Colitis ulcerosa-Kranken. Langenbecks Arch. Chir. 293: 558–570, 1960
Reifferscheid, M.: Pathogenesis of sigmoid diverticulitis and indications for resection. Langenbecks Arch. Chir. 318: 134–160, 1967
Reynolds, E.O.: Carcinoma of the colon in a child. Brit. med. J. 5254: 749–750, 1961
Reynolds, R.M., F.Wietersen, R.P.Reynolds: Intramural diverticulitis. Ann. Surg. 151: 251–254, 1960
Rice, R.P.: Plain abdominal film roentgenographic diagnosis of ulcerative disease of the colon. Amer. J. Roentgenol. 104: 544–550, 1968
Ricketts, W.E., J.B.Kirsner, W.L.Palmer: Chronic nonspecific ulcerative colitis. Gastroenterology 10: 1–15, 1948
Rider, J.A., J.B.Kirsner, H.C.Moeller, W.L.Palmer: Polyps of the colon and rectum; their incidence and relationship to carcinoma. Amer. J. Med. 16: 555–564, 1954
Riederer, J.: Zur Abgrenzung der Endometriose gegen das Karzinom des Dickdarms. Radiol. Clin. (Basel) 31: 48–54, 1962
Rigler, L.G., L.G.Eriksen: Benign tumors of stomach: observations on their incidence and malignant degeneration. Radiology 26: 6–15, 1936
Ripstein, C.B.: Perforation of colon in ulcerative colitis. Amer. Surg. 140: 872–874, 1954
Ritvo, M., C.Litner: Roentgen manifestations of primary amyloidosis of the colon. Amer. J. Roentgenol. 89: 760–765, 1963
Ritvo, M., I.A.Shauffer: Gastrointestinal x-ray diagnosis. Kimpton, London 1952
Robertson, H.E.: Polyps of the colon and their possible significance, Bull. Amer. Soc. Cancer. 16: 6–7, 1934
Robinson, J.M.: Detection of small lesions of the large bowel; barium enema versus double contrast. Calif. Med. 81: 321–324, 1954
Rodkey, G.V., G.Herman: Diverticulitis of the right colon. Amer. J. Surg. 101: 61–65, 1961
de Rojas, J.F., H.S.Irons jr: Diverticulosis of the appendix. Arch. Surg. 96: 429–432, 1968
Root, J.C., C.M.Greenwald: Double contrast study of colon; Routine lateral recumbent view. Radiology 63: 241–245, 1954
Rosenqvist, H., R.Lagercrantz, H.Öhrling, N.Edling: Ulcerative colitis and carcinoma coli. Lancet 1: 906–908, 1959
Rosenzweig, J., A.Horwitz: Adenomatous tumors of the colon and rectum: the importance of early detection and treatment. Amer. Surg. 24: 515–520, 1958
Ross, S.T.: Granulomatous colitis. Surgery 58: 357–363, 1965
Ross, S.T., E.J.Eddy: Massive hemorrhage from diverticulitis. Dis. Colon Rect. 3: 441–445, 1960
Roth, J.L.A., A.Valdes-Dapena, G.N.Stein, H.L. Bockus: Toxic megacolon in ulcerative colitis. Gastroenterology 37: 239–255, 1959
Rowden, W.H.: Diverticulitis with particular reference to its diagnosis by radiology. Brit. med. J. 1: 381–383, 1930
Rowe, R.J.: Dilatation of the colon (toxic megacolon) in acute fulminating ulcerative colitis. Dis. Colon Rect. 6: 23–36, 1963
Rudhe, U.: Roentgenologic examination of rectum in ulcerative colitis. Acta paediat. (Uppsala) 49: 859–867, 1960
Rudhe, U., T.E.Keats: Granulomatous colitis in children. Radiology 84: 24–32, 1965
Runyeon, F.G.: Surgical management of chronic ulcerative colitis. Dis. Colon Rect. 2: 362–365, 1959
Rüttiman, A., M.S.Del Buono, F.Ensesa: Radiological colon examination, according to the double contrast method. Med. mundi 7: 98–106, 1961
Ryan, P.: Solitary sigmoid diverticulitis. Brit. J. Surg. 52: 85–89, 1965

Salvati, E., H.H.Bong, C.F.Varga: Massive hemorrhage from colonic diverticula caused by arterial erosion: a practical theory of its mechanism and causation. Dis. Colon Rect. 10: 129–135, 1967
Santosh, C., P.Munkerjee, K.Bery: Segmental tuberculosis of the colon. (A report of ten cases). Clin. Radiol. 22: 104–109, 1971
Sawyer, H.F.: Polypi of rectum. Amer. J. Surg. 50: 657–660, 1940
Sawyer, K.C., R.B.Sawyer, H.U.Waggener: The pathogenesis of diverticulosis coli. Dis. Colon Rect. 12: 49–57, 1969
Scarborough, R.A.: The significance of rectal bleeding in diverticulosis and diverticulitis of the colon. Dis. Colon Rect. 1: 49–52, 1958
Scarborough, R.A.: The relationship between polyps and carcinoma of the colon and rectum. Dis. Colon Rect. 3: 336–342, 1960
Scarborough, R.A.: Adenomatous polyps of the rectum and colon. Dis. Colon Rect. 8: 85–96, 1965
Scarborough, R.A., R.R.Klein: Polypoid lesions of colon and rectum. Amer. J. Surg. 76: 723–727, 1948
Schachter, H., M.J.Goldstein et al.: Ulcerative and granulomatous colitis – Validity of differential diagnostic criteria. A study of 100 patients treated by total colectomy. Ann. intern. Med. 72: 841–851, 1970
Schachter, H., M.J.Goldstein, J.B.Kirsner: Toxic dilatation complicating Crohn's disease of the colon. Gastroenterology 53: 136–142, 1967
Schapira, A., J.J.Leichtling, B.S.Wolf, R.H.Marshak, H.J.Janowitz: Diverticulitis of the cecum and right colon: clinical and radiographic features. Amer. J. digest. Dis. 3: 351–383, 1958
Schapiro, S.: The occurrence of proctologic disorders in infancy and childhood, a statistical review of 2,700 cases. Gastroenterology 15: 653–666, 1950
Scharer, L.L., H.J.Burhenne: Megacolon. A nonspecific sign. Clinical and roentgenological differentiation. Radiol. Clin. (Basel) 34: 236–246, 1965
Schaupp, W.C., D.M.Gallagher, R.A.Scarborough: Regional enteritis. Dis. Colon Rect. 10: 6–12, 1967
Schexnayder, E.A.: The unstable colon: its role as a precursor to diverticulitis. New Orleans med. surg. J. 99: 496–499, 1947
Schibalski, H.: Die konservative Heilung der Colitis ulcerosa im Röntgenbild. Fortschr. Röntgenstr. 96: 399–410, 1962
Schilla, F.W.: Carcinoma in a rectal polyp; report of a case in infancy. Amer. J. Surg. 88: 759–760, 1954
Schmidt, G.: Crohn's disease of the colon and diverticulitis. Med. J. Aust. 2: 1253–1258, 1969
Schmidt, G.T., J.E.Lennard-Jones, B.C.Morson, A.C. Young: Crohn's disease of the colon and its distinction from diverticulitis. Gut 9: 7–16, 1968
Schmieden, V., H.Westhues: Zur Klinik und Pathologie der Dickdarmpolypen und deren klinischen und pathologisch-anatomischen Beziehungen zum Dickdarmkarzinom. Dtsch. Z. Chir. 202: 1–124, 1927
Schofield, P.F.: Some aspects of Crohn's disease. Dis. Colon Rect. 10: 262–266, 1967
Schofield, P.F., H.Fox: The diagnosis of Crohn's disease of the colon; a clinico-pathological study. Brit. J. Surg. 54: 307–311, 1967

Schreiber, H.W.: Neue Gesichtspunkte zur Divertikulitis des Dickdarms. Dtsch. med. Wschr. 90: 1998–2002, 1965

Schwartz, S., S.Boley, J.Lash, V.Sternhill: Roentgenologic aspects of reversible vascular occlusion of the colon and its relationship to ulcerative colitis. Radiology 80: 625–635, 1963

Scott, W.G.: Cancer of the colon and its early diagnosis. J. Iowa St. med. Soc. 40: 513–517, 1950

Seaman, W.B.: Disease of the colon. New concepts, old problems. Radiology 100: 251–269, 1971

Senturia, H.R., S.M.Wald: Ulcerative disease of the intestinal tract proximal to partially obstructing lesions: roentgen appearance. Amer. J. Roentgenol. 99: 45–51, 1967

Shaiken, J.: Diverticulitis and carcinoma of the sigmoid colon. Gastroenterology 27: 67–74, 1954

Shapira, A., J.J.Leichtling, B.S.Wolf, R.H.Marshak, H. D.Janowitz: Diverticulitis of cecum and right colon, clinical and radiographic features. Amer. J. dig. Dis. 3, 351–383, 1958

Sharpe, M., R.Golden: End to end anastomosis of the colon following resection. Amer. J. Roentgenol. 64: 769–777, 1950

Siegal, H.A.: Endometriosis simulating carcinoma of the colon. Amer. J. Proctol. 20: 192–201, 1969

Simon, M., J.H.Shapiro, J.G.Parker, C.J.Shein, B. Weingarten: The diagnosis and treatment of dilatation of the colon in severe colitis. A diagnostic roentgen sign. Amer. J. Roentgenol. 87: 655–659, 1962

Simpkins, K.C., G.W.Stevenson: The modified Malmö double contrast barium enema in colitis. An assement of its accuracy in reflecting sigmoidoscopic findings. Brit. J. Radiol. 45: 486–492, 1972

Simpkins, K.C., A.C.Young: The differential diagnosis of large bowel strictures. Clin. Radiol. 22: 449–457, 1971

Singleton, A.C., M.R.Hall: Diverticulitis of the sigmoid colon. A radiological study. Canad. med. Ass. J. 37: 525–530, 1937

Sjögren, S.: Morbus Crohn. Svensk för. med. Radiol. Stockholm 1969

Slack, W.W.: Diverticula of the colon and their relation to the muscle layers and blood vessels. Gastroenterology 39: 708–712, 1960

Slack, W.W.: The anatomy, pathology, and some clinical features of diverticulitis of the colon. Brit. J. Surg. 50: 185–190, 1962

Slack, W.W.: Bowel muscle in diverticular disease. Gut 7: 668–670, 1966

Slaney, G., B.N.Brooke: Cancer in ulcerative colitis. Lancet 2: 694–698, 1959

Smedal, M.J.: Polyps of the colon from radiologic viewpoint. Surg. Clin. N. Amer. 21: 845–853, 1941

Smith, C.C., W.R.Christensen: The incidence of colonic diverticulosis. Amer. J. Roentgenol. 82: 996–999, 1959

Smith, M.: Chronic ulcerative colitis with pseudopolyposis. Dis. Colon Rect. 9: 173–175, 1966

Spjuth, H.J., D.E.Perkins: Endometriosis of the sigmoid colon and rectum. Amer. J. Roentgenol. 82: 1070–1075, 1959

Spratt, J.S., L.V.Ackerman: Relationship of size of colonic tumors to their cellular composition and biological behavior. Surg. Forum 10: 56–61, 1960

Spratt, J.S., L.V.Ackerman: Growth of a colonic adenocarcinoma. Amer. Surg. 27: 23–28, 1961

Spratt, J.S., L.V.Ackerman: Small primary adenocarcinomas of colon and rectum. J. Amer. med. Ass. 179: 337–346, 1962

Spratt, J.S., L.V.Ackerman, C.D.Moyer: Relationship of polyps of the colon to colonic cancer. Ann. Surg. 148: 682–698, 1958

Spriggs, E.I.: Diverticulitis. Brit. med. J. 2: 569–574, 1929

Spriggs, E.I., O.A.Marxer: Multiple diverticula of the colon. Lancet 1: 1067–1074, 1927

Stanley, P., I.K.Fry, A.M.Dawson, N.Dyer: Radiological signs of ulcerative colitis and Crohn's disease of the colon. Clin. Radiol. 22: 434–442, 1971

de Stefano, L.V., D.Horwath: Studio clinico e radiologico sulla polyposi del colon. Gazz. int. Med. Chir. 64: 2816–2833, 1959

Stein, G.N., R.H.Roy, A.K.Finkelstein: Roentgen changes in ulcerative colitis. Sem. Roentgenol. 3: 3–26, 1928

Sternberg, A.: Diverticulitis of the colon with special attention to the x-ray picture. Harefuah 60: 247, 251, 1961

Stevenson, C.A.: Symposium on gastrointestinal surgery; technic of the double contrast examination of the colon. Surg. Clin. N. Amer. 32: 1531–1537, 1952

Stevenson, C.A.: The development of the colon examination. Amer. J. Roentgenol. 71: 385–397, 1954

Stevenson, C.A., M.Wilson: Double contrast manifestation of nonpolypoid colon diseases. Tex. St. J. Med. 48: 826–831, 1952

Stevenson, C.A., M.Wilson: Indications for double contrast colon examination. Amer. J. Roentgenol. 71: 398–403, 1954

Stewart, M.J.: Precancerous lesions of the alimentary tract. Lancet 2: 669–675, 1931

Stierlin, E.: Die Radiographie in der Diagnostik der Ileozoekaltuberkulose und anderer Krankheiten des Dickdarms. Münch. med. Wschr. 58: 1231–1235, 1911

Storrs, R.C., R.A.Hoeckelman: Acute regional enteritis in children. New Engl. J. Med. 248: 320–322, 1953

Stout, A.P.: Tumors of the colon and rectum. In Turell, R. editor: Diseases of the colon and anorectum, Vol. I. Saunders, Philadelphia 1959

Straubinger, C.A.: Villous papilloma of the colon and rectum. Dis. Colon Rect. 1: 283–289, 1958

Stuart, H., E.B.Castro: Papillary adenomas (villous tumors). A review of 215 cases. Dis. Colon Rect. 14: 267–280, 1971

Sundberg, C.A.: Neuere Erfahrungen über Colondivertikel. Nord. med. T. 2, 504–511, 1931

Sunderland, D.A., G.E.Binkley: Papillary adenomas of the large intestine, clinical and morphological study of 48 cases. Cancer 1: 184–207, 1948

Susman, W.: Polypi coli. J. Path. Bact. 35: 29–33, 1932

Sutcliffe, J.: Crohn's disease of the colon. Brit. J. Radiol. 36: 27–32, 1963

Swartz, N., T.Ernberg: Cancer coli in cases of colitis ulcerosa. Acta med. scand. 135: 444–447, 1949

Swenson, P.C., R.Wigh: The role of the roentgenologist in diagnosis of polypoid disease of the colon. Amer. J. Roentgenol. 59: 108–121, 1948

Swinton, N.W.: Significance of mucosal polyps of colon and rectum. Surg. Clin. N. America 27: 675–680, 1947

Swinton, N.W., A.D.Haug: Frequency of precancerous lesions in rectum and colon. Lahey Clin. Bull. 5: 84–88, 1947

Swinton, N.W., J.C.Snow: Treatment of rectal and colonic polyps showing early malignant change. Dis. Colon Rect. 3: 113–116, 1960

Swinton, N.W., S.Warren: Polyps of colon and rectum and their relation to malignancy. J. Amer. med. Ass. 113: 1927–1933, 1939

Theander, G., L.Wehlin: Deformation of the rectosigmoid junction in peritoneal carcinomatosis. Acta radiol. (Stockh) 55: 241–248, 1961

Theander, G., L.Wehlin: Die Schrumpf-Deformität des Dickdarmes im Grenzgebiet zwischen Rectum und Sigma. Radiologe 2: 100–107, 1962

Theander, G., L. Wehlin, P. Langeland: Deformation of the recto-sigmoid junction in peritoneal carcinomatosis. Acta radiol. (Stockh) 1: 1071–1076, 1963
Thompson, J.W.: Acute sigmoid diverticulitis. J. int. Coll. Surg. 17: 52–64, 1952
Thompson, J.E., R.L. Pinck: Adenomatous polyps of the large bowel; their significance to the surgeon. Amer. Surg. 22: 964–974, 1956
Tondreau, R.L.: Multiple primary carcinoma of the large intestine. Amer. J. Roentgenol. 71: 794–807, 1954
Tucker: In discussion W.J. Martin Sth. med. J. (Bgham, Ala) 33: 428–432, 1940
Turek, R.E., W.C. Davis, W.J. Wilson, R.O. Olson: The roentgenographic diagnosis of villous tumors of the colon. Amer. J. Roentgenol. 113: 349–351, 1971
Turell, R.: Colonic adenomas. Amer. J. Surg. 76: 783–789, 1948
Turell, R.: Adenomas of the colon and rectum in children. Surg. Clin. N. Amer. 40: 985–997, 1960
Turell, R., H.R. Brodman: Adenomas of colon and rectum. In: Diseases of the colon and anorectum hrsg. von R. Turell. Saunders, Philadelphia 1959
Turell, R., A. de L. Maynard: Adenomas of the rectum and colon in juvenile patients. J. Amer. med. Ass. 161: 57–60, 1956
Turell, R., A.A. Pommeranz, R. Paradny, L.A. Vallecillo: Adenomas of the colon and rectum with special emphasis on therapy. Surg. Clin. N. Amer. 35: 1259–1275, 1955
Turnbull, R.B.: Carcinoma in polyps of the colon and rectum. A study of 86 treated patients. Dis. Colon Rect. 1: 44–48, 1958

Valdes-Dapena, A., W.J. Beckfield: Adenomatous polyps of the large intestine: pathology and histogenesis. Gastroenterology 32: 452–461, 1957
Versé, M.: Über die Entstehung, den Bau und Wachstum der Polypen, Adenom und Karzinom des Magendarmkanals. Arb. path. anat. Bakt 1: 5, 1908

Walker, F.C., G.T. Curtis: Irreversible changes of ulcerative colitis. Brit. med. J. 1: 414–416, 1965
Walske, B.P., J.W. Hamilton, P. Kirsner: From benign polyp to carcinoma. Ann. Surg. 70: 318–322, 1955
Wangensteen, O.H.: Cancer of the colon and rectum. Wis. med. J. 48: 591–597, 1949
Warren, S., S.C. Sommers: Cicatrizing enteritis (regional ileitis) as pathologic entity: analysis of 120 cases. Amer. J. Path. 24: 475–502, 1948
Warren, S., S.C. Sommers: Pathology of regional ileitis and ulcerative colitis. J. Amer. med. Ass. 154: 189–193, 1954
Watkinson, G., H. Thompson, J.C. Goligher: Rightsided or segmental ulcerative colitis. Brit. J. Surg. 47: 337–351, 1960
Weber, H.M.: Roentgenologic demonstration of polypoid lesions and polyposis of large intestine. Amer. J. Roentgenol. 25: 577–589, 1931
Weber, H.M.: Roentgenologic aspects of polypoid lesions, polyposis and polypoidosis. Proc. Mayo Clin. 15: 103–105, 1940
Weber, H.M.: Significance of intestinal polypoid lesion. J. Amer. med. Ass. 142: 693–697, 1950
Weber, H.M.: The diagnosis of early intestinal cancer. Amer. J. Roentgenol. 64: 929–937, 1950
Weingarten, M., R. Turell: Carcinomatous mucosal excrescenses of the rectum. J. Amer. med. Ass. 149: 1467–1468, 1952
Welch, C.E.: Diverticulitis of the colon. Amer. J. Gastroent. 29: 374–383, 1958
Welch, C.E., J.B. McKittrik, G. Behringer: Polyps of the rectum and colon and their relation to cancer. New Engl. J. Med. 247: 959–965, 1952
Welch, J.S., M.B. Dockerty: Villous carcinomas of the colon. Dis. Colon Rect. 1: 251–261, 1958
Welin, S.: Clysodrast. Observanda medica, Ferrosan Malmö 1955
Welin, S.: Zur Darstellung der Kolonpolypen mit der Doppelkontrastmethode. Fortschr. Röntgenstr. 82: 341–344, 1955
Welin, S.: Röntgendiagnostik von Kolonpolypen. In: Röntgendiagnostik, Ergebnisse 1952–1956, hrsg. v. H.R. Schinz, R. Glauner, E. Uehlinger. Thieme, Stuttgart 1957 (S. 439–454)
Welin, S.: Modern trends in diagnostic roentgenology of colon. Brit. J. Radiol. 31: 453–464, 1958
Welin, S.: Über moderne röntgenologische Dickdarmdiagnostik unter besonderer Berücksichtigung der Doppelkontrastmethode. Münch. med. Wschr. 100: 1142–1144, 1958
Welin, S.: Siebenjährige Erfahrung mit der Doppelkontrastmethode. Radiol. diagn. (Berl.) 2: 173–182, 1961
Welin, S.: Über die Differentialdiagnose gutartiger und bösartiger Colonerkrankungen vom röntgenologischen Standpunkt. Langenbecks Arch. Chir. 31: 376–381, 1962
Welin, S.: Über die röntgenologische Untersuchung des Dickdarms mit der Doppelkontrastmethode. Die Malmömodifikation. Radiologe 2: 87–100, 1962
Welin, S.: Erfahrungen von 20.000 Untersuchungen des Colons mit der Doppelkontrastmethode. Weltkongreß für Gastroenterologie II: 811–814, 1962
Welin, S.: Die Doppelkontrastuntersuchung des Dickdarms. Röntgenpraxis 16: 69–75, 1963
Welin, S.: Technik und Ergebnisse des Doppelkontrastverfahrens des Colon. Z. Gastroent. 1: 63–69, 1963
Welin, S.: The double contrast examination of the colon. T. Gastro-ent. 6: 605–614, 1963
Welin, S.: Advances in roentgen diagnosis of ulcerative colitis. Acta chir. scand. 125: 482–484, 1963
Welin, S.: Double contrast examination of the large intestine in children. Ann. Radiol. 7: 406–411, 1964
Welin, S.: Results of the Malmö technique of colon examination. J. Amer. med. Ass. 199: 369–371, 1967
Welin, S.: Polyps in colon-rectum and cancer. Radiological diagnosis. In: Thule Intern. Symposium, Cancer and Ageing. 253–257. Nordiska Bokhandeln, Stockholm 1968
Welin, S.: The radiological detection of early carcinoma and pre-malignant lesions of the colon and rectum. J. Roy. Coll. Surg. Edinb. 14: 278–286, 1969
Welin, S.: The technical approach in the study of the large bowel with particular emphasis on the examinations for polyps. Prgr. pediat. Radiol. 2: 52–64, 1969
Welin, S.: The radiological detection of early carcinoma. J. belge Radiol. 54: 21–30, 1971
Welin, S.: Examination and cleansing of the large bowel. J. belge Radiol. 54: 1–6, 1971
Welin, S., L. Andrén: Colon and rectum. In: Lehrbuch der Röntgendiagnostik, hrsg. von H.R. Schinz, W.E. Baensch, W. Frommhold, R. Glauner, E. Uehlinger, J. Wellauer. Thieme, Stuttgart 1965 (S. 329–364
Welin, S., F. Brahme: The double contrast method in ulcerative colitis. Acta radiol. (Stockh) 55: 257–271, 1961
Welin, S., P. Lörinc: Das Röntgenbild des villösen Tumors im Bereich des Colons. Radiologe 2: 107–112, 1962
Welin, S., G. Welin: A new pathognomonic roentgenologic sign of regional ileitis (Crohn's disease). Dis. Colon Rect. 16: 473–478, 1973
Welin, S., G. Welin: Ein "neues pathognomonisches, differentialdiagnostisches Zeichen zwischen Colitis ulcerosa und Crohnscher Krankheit. Kongreßbericht 1973. Fortschr. Röntgenstr, Beiheft 1974

Welin, S., J. Youker: Differentiation of true polypoid tumors of the colon from extraneous material. A new roentgen sign. Radiology 84: 610–615, 1967
Welin, S., J. Youker: Colonic polyps. In: Alimentary tract. Editors Margulis, A.R., H.J. Burhenne. Mosby, St. Louis 1967 (S. 811–833)
Welin, S., G. Welin, T. Åberg: Klyxray; a new preparation for excessive emptying of the colon. Brit. J. Radiol. 43: 744–746, 1970
Welin, S., J. Youker, J.S. Spratt: The rates and patterns of growth of 375 tumors of the large intestine and rectum, observed serially by the double contrast enema study (Malmö technique). Amer. J. Roentgenol. 90: 673–687, 1963
Wheat jr, M.W., L.V. Ackerman: Villous adenomas the large intestine. Clinicopathologic evaluation of 50 cases of villous adenomas with emphasis on treatment. Ann. Surg. 147: 476–487, 1958
Wietersen, F.K.: High kilovoltage method of investigation of the colon as a routine roentgenological procedure. Amer. J. Roentgenol. 77: 690–699, 1957
Wigh, R., P.C. Swenson: Roentgenologic aspects of diverticulitis and its complications. Amer. J. Surg. 82: 587–596, 1951
Wilcox jr, H.R., J.L. Beattie: Carcinoma complicating ulcerative colitis during childhood. Amer. J. clin. Path. 26: 778–786, 1956
Williams, I.: Changing emphasis in diverticular disease of the colon. Brit. J. Radiol. 36: 393–406, 1963
Williams, I.: The resemblance of diverticular disease of the colon to a myostatic contracture. Brit. J. Radiol. 38: 437–443, 1965
Williams, I.: Innominate grooves in the surface of mucosa. Radiology 84: 877–880, 1965
Williams, I.: Mass movements (mass peristalsis) and diverticular disease of the colon. Brit. J. Radiol. 40: 2–14, 1967
Williams, I.: Diverticular disease of the colon without diverticula. Radiology 89: 401–412, 1967
Williams jr, L.F., M.A. Bosniak, J. Wittenberg et al.: Ischemic colitis. Amer. J. Surg. 117: 254–264, 1969
Winblad, S., S. Frieberg: Observations on the pathology of polyps of the colon. Acta path. microbiol. scand., suppl. 111: 89–92, 1956
Wolf, B.S.: Roentgen findings in diverticulitis of the right side of colon. J. Mt. Sinai Hosp. 23: 697–710, 1956
Wolf, B.S.: Roentgen diagnosis of villous tumors of the colon. Amer. J. Roentgenol. 84: 1093–1104, 1960
Wolf, B.S., R.H. Marshak: "Toxic" segmental dilatation of the colon during the course of fulminating ulcerative colitis: roentgen findings. Amer. J. Roentgenol. 82: 985–995, 1959
Wolf, B.S., R.H. Marshak: Granulomatous colitis. (Crohn's disease of the colon). Amer. J. Roentgenol. 88: 662–670, 1962
Wolf, B.S., R.H. Marshak: Linitis plastica or diffusely infiltrating type of carcinoma of the colon. Radiology 81: 502–507, 1963
Wolf, B.S., M.T. Khilnani, R.H. Marshak: Diverticulosis and diverticulitis; roentgen findings and their interpretation. Amer. J. Roentgenol. 77: 726–743, 1957
Wolf, B.S., M. Melamed, R. Turell: Juvenile polyps (Adenomas) of the colon – clinical and roentgen features. J. Mt. Sinai Hosp. 28: 327–333, 1961
Wright, V., G. Watkinson: Sacro-iliitis and ulcerative colitis. Brit. med. J. 5463: 675–680, 1965

Yaker, D.N.: Carcinoid of the rectum. Clinics 3: 1055–1058, 1944
Yarnis, H., B.B. Crohn: Segmental (ulcerative) colitis. Gastroenterology 38: 721–728, 1960
Yates, C.W.: Double contrast studies of the colon: polyps in children. Sth. med. J. (Bgham, Ala.) 46: 315–319, 1953
Yates, C.W., R.D. Moreton, E.M. Cooper: Double contrast studies of the colon with special reference to preparation and fictitious polyps. Radiology 55: 539–544, 1950
Youker, J.E., S. Welin: Differentiation of true polypoid tumors of the colon from extraneous material; a new roentgen sign. Radiology 84: 610–615, 1965
Youker, J.E., S. Welin, G. Main: Computer analysis in the differentiation of benign and malignant polypoid lesions of the colon. Radiology 90: 794–797, 1967
Young, A.C.: Surgical management of diverticulitis. Dis. Colon Rect. 8: 165–174, 1965
Young, A.C.: Diverticular disease. In: B.C. Morson (Ed.): Tutorials in postgraduate medicine, London 1969
Young, B.R., R.L. Scanlan: Roentgen demonstration and significance of the pedicle in polypoid tumors of the alimentary tract. Amer. J. Roentgenol. 68: 894–899, 1952

Zarate, V.E., W. Koch: The radiological aspect of aspecific ulcerative colitis. Rev. med. Valparaiso 8: 103–108, 1955
Zdansky, E., A. Werthemann: Die Entwicklung und der Verlauf der Diverticulitis coli im Röntgenbild und dessen anatomische Grundlagen. Med. Welt (Stuttgart) 20: 1119–1122, 1965

Index